Fun to Be Fit

Books in Print
BY Marie Chapian
  Help Me Remember . . . Help Me Forget (formerly *The Emancipation of
  Robert Sadler*)
  Of Whom the World Was Not Worthy
  Free to Be Thin
  In the Morning of My Life (the story of singer Tom Netherton)
  Telling Yourself the Truth (with Dr. William Backus)
  Escape From Rage
  Fun to Be Fit

Marie Chapian

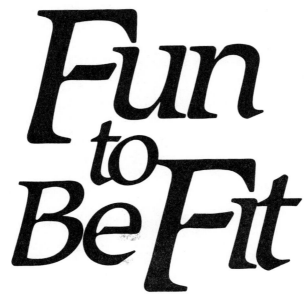

Fun to Be Fit

Staying in Shape
With a Life-Changing
Exercise Plan

Fleming H. Revell Company
Old Tappan, New Jersey

Library of Congress Cataloging in Publication Data

Chapian, Marie.
    Fun to be fit.

    Bibliography: p.
    1. Exercise.   2. Physical fitness.
3. Exercise—religious aspects—Christianity.
4. Physical fitness—Religious aspects—
Christianity.   5. Christian life—1960–
I. Title.
RA781.C473   1983   613.7'1   82-13265
ISBN 0-8007-1317-6

TO
Christa
and
Liza

Special thanks and a David Dance to these who helped
so unselfishly in preparing this book:
Cathy Slater
Tina Urnezis
Jenny Offner
Mom
Great-Uncle Fred
my wonderful staff, students, counselees, and friends
at the Christian Center for Counseling and Fitness in
San Diego, California
Fritz Ridenour, my friend and editor
and special leaps and claps for the
Revell production department
headed by Joseph A. Repole. i love you.

CONTENTS

i think of You, Lord,
       walking this earth on dusty roads
       beneath frowning skies,
                              and i imagine
                              Your stride,
Your strong stride,
        Your strong
Self.
       You told us
       we are the temples
       of God,
that we are His treasure,
His *best* creation,
              and You, the Cornerstone,
              our model, hero, savior and Lord,
              walked the cold, crabbed, splenetic
              earth
lovely, fit and wholesome:
       Perfect.

                   i want only to (in
                   every way)

be like
You
, especially in the teeth of a rising storm
              of temptation
              to choose
                         less,
i want to be
   the sweet fruit
of Your soul's anguish;
     O love,
i want to satisfy
   the purpose for
Your life
                   when You gave Your fitness
                   to the Cross
                   meant
                   for me.

marie jordan chapian
La Jolla, California
February 1982

Yet it was our grief he bore,
    our sorrows that weighed him down
    . . . he was wounded and bruised for
our sins. He was
    chastised that we might
        have peace;
he was lashed—and we were
            healed!
. . . But when his soul
    has been made an offering
        for sin,
then he shall have
          a multitude of
          children,
          many heirs.
He shall live again
      and God's program shall prosper
      in his hands.
    And when he sees all that is accomplished
by
the anguish of his soul,
he shall be
satisfied. . . .*

                  The Prophet Isaiah, son of Amoz
                            Judah
                            712 B.C.

* Isaiah 53:4–11 TLB

PREFACE

That person grinning away at you on the cover of this book is none other than an ex out-of-shape chubbette who hated any exercise more taxing than plumping a pillow or opening and closing a refrigerator door. If I touched my toes once a week, I thought I was being athletic. I was—if you'll pardon the expression—lazy. Maybe you're a person like I was, who considered pressing the buttons on the blender physical activity, and polishing pots and pans worthy of a two-week rest in bed.

Mind you, I worked hard, though. I mean, it was nothing for me to work around the clock on a manuscript deadline, and I traveled thousands of miles a year as a speaker. I mean, I *worked.* But I discovered it's possible to work yourself into a dither and be lazy at the same time. It was my body that told me that. I overheard it one morning as I was getting dressed. "Help!" it screamed as I tried to squeeze into a new dress. "You'll never be able to sit down in this dress." It went on to say, "And furthermore, it's not decent to wear something that looks painted on!" Would you believe it? Even those blatant messages didn't quite reach me. I just changed dresses.

My body would tell me how exhausted it was and I would ignore those promptings, too. For example, let me tell you about my Great-Uncle Fred who is eighty-some years old. (He admits to eighty, anyhow.) Uncle Fred is in shape. He has a stomach so flat you could use him for a ruler. Charming, energetic, strong, his only complaint in life is that he doesn't see as well as he used to. Many a time I have huffed and puffed alongside him, vainly trying to keep up as he climbed the steps of his home in La Jolla, California.

One day when I went to visit Uncle Fred, after groaning up his steps, I found him doing sit-ups on his slant board in the living room.

"Good heavens, what are you doing, Uncle Fred? Do you want to *hurt* yourself?"

He graciously invited me to have a seat, and went on counting. "Ninety-two—ninety-three—"

"I'll call the paramedics," I stammered.

"Don't be silly—ninety-seven—I'm *fine!*"

"Not for you, for *me!*" I gasped. "I think I pulled something closing the door."

I was starting to get the message. Uncle Fred's example was convicting me of my own out-of-shape condition. Not with words, mind you. It was those barbells in the corner of his studio. Unfair, I thought, that an eighty-some-year-old person should be able to sling those things around like chicken bones when I couldn't even close a door without dislocating something.

A few days and several granola bars and strawberry yogurts later, my young daughters and I were walking past a large plate-glass window on the campus of the University of California. I saw my reflection and stopped in my tracks. "Look at this, would you!" I chuckled. "Here's one of those trick mirrors."

My children looked puzzled. "What are you talking about, Mom?"

"Well, just look! I mean, this window makes me look positively *chubby.* Ha ha."

Silence.

I continued my amusing observation. "Isn't this funny, girls? I look like a *blimp.* Ha ha."

(Nervous throat clearing and obvious nonamused reaction from children.)

"This window must be made of cheap glass or something, huh? Uh, girls?"

My eldest daughter, age fourteen and thin as a fence post, said in her inimitable soft way of saying hard things, "Mom . . . will you look at *my* reflection in the same window?"

"Sure!" (Sudden apprehension.) "There you are, thin as a—oh, dear."

Number Two daughter, age twelve, spoke: "And now look at *my* reflection, Mom."

An accurate duplication of the tiny, bony creature she was stared back at me. I looked from one to the other, noting painfully two skinny-legged girls who looked exactly like themselves. The chubbette in the middle had to be none other than *moi.*

"I'll never eat again," I gasped. "Never. Never. Christa, tape my lips." I grabbed Number One daughter by the lean arm. "Promise me, if you ever see a fork aimed at my mouth, you'll release the house alarm. Promise!" Number Two stood nervously poking her toe at the ground. I threw my arms around her narrow shoulders. "My goodness! You have a *flabby* mother! Poor, deprived child!" I was nearly hysterical now. "Oh, Liza, I give you my word. I will make it up to you—somehow—someday!"

I was utterly undone. I felt bad enough that my eighty-some-year-old Great-Uncle Fred was more fit than I, but this was just too much.

I kept my promise. In four months I lost thirty-five pounds, resisting the temptation to pray for a bona fide case of anorexia nervosa. (Something I once suffered with, by the way—an awful way to go.) And I exercised! For a fat, lazy

person it was a miracle. Finally I learned the secret of how to set the *real* me free from the flabby person in the window that day.

My body and I are a team now. I am healthy, energetic, in control of myself, and I don't ever want to go back to what I saw that awful day on campus. I feel as though God has given me an entirely new life, inside and out. It's incredible.

I discovered that getting in shape was actually *fun.* I devised a program that was exciting instead of boring. While developing this program, I discovered a power I hadn't really tapped before. I had been thin before in my life and I had also been in shape before in my life. I had been a ballet dancer in my early years, and had trained diligently, but at this point in my life, I feel more in control of myself and my body than I did even when I was a professional dancer.

The program you are about to begin will not only reshape your body but it will also reshape your entire life. I believe it will change your life forever. You will take off weight, keep it off, and you'll learn the exercises your body needs to get in shape and stay in shape. You'll learn what a really strong, beautiful person you really are.

This is not a thirty-day crash program. Those programs only leave you sore and hungry, anyhow. I have been on thirty-day crash programs and sure enough, I crashed. This is a lifelong plan that will change you forever because you will be plugging into the power of God. He will become your ability to accomplish a new healthy you.

God *wants* you to be healthy and strong. Can you imagine Him creating you in His image as a sickly, overweight, weak, and flabby person? Please, now!

My program will not give you overnight results, but lasting results. Take time. We are after a Total You, a person who, body, soul, and spirit, is totally in charge because of the dynamic power of God within you.

You're going to be a happier person on this program, I guarantee you. You're going to learn an exercise program I call "Blessercize," aerobics, and an aerobic routine called the David Dance.

I have never heard one person say how unhappy he or she was to look great and feel great, have you? Get ready to say good-bye to that weight problem, those flabby legs, and that spare-tire tummy. Say good-bye to weakness, past failures, and dimpled thighs. You may be out of shape today, but there's no reason for you to be out of shape tomorrow.

Get ready to have one of the greatest times of your life. God wants to bless you, body and all!

Love, your friend,
Marie

115 pounds
61 resting pulse rate

Fun to Be Fit

1

Fun to Be Fit

Your Fun to Be Fit program is not like any other program you've tried before. I believe it was God who created your body, and so it should be God who blesses it and keeps it running in optimum condition. *He* has got to be at the center of every workout you do. He's the one who figured out your cardiovascular system, your lymph system, your basal metabolism, muscle groupings, tendons, tissues, circulatory system, nervous system, bone formation, blood, and brain. Since your body is His invention, He knows best how it ought to be maintained. You will do this program *with* Him, not apart from Him while begging His distant and ever-out-of-reach help with your painful labors. You'll experience the Lord alongside you and within you as your body becomes His instrument to revitalize and breathe new life and energy into. He will guide and help and bless your *entire* being: body, soul, and spirit.

Your Beginning

When beginning any new program, no matter what it is, there is a point when you must make up your mind to dedicate yourself to it with an honest and dedicated purpose. No matter how lazy, fat, old, young, or weak you are, you can be healthier, happier, and filled with more energy if you will commit yourself to a "fit for a lifetime" program.

I know people who hate the very words *physical fitness*. It sounds like too much work for them. But physical fitness doesn't have to be tedious work! God doesn't want you worn out, miserable, aching, and hobbling around in pain after sporadic attempts at exercise. I like what Deborah Szekely Mazzanti, founder of the famous exclusive spa the Golden Door, says: "Exercise can be dull, therefore I must help make it irresistible." This fabulous spa where the stars go to shape up runs under the firm belief that most health regimens fail because they lack the element of enjoyment.

The Fun to Be Fit program I am sharing with you here has been, for me, far *more* than enjoyable. It has changed my life and given me an inner thrill that has gone deeper than happiness. The program is changing many others' lives, too. I pray it will change yours.

There is one prerequisite, and that is, at this beginning point, you ask yourself this question: *Do I want to be healthy?* If you can answer yes to that question, you are ready for the next step, which is to ask yourself if you want to be committed to be healthy.

For too long our physical selves have been disassociated from our spiritual selves. We've been partial Christians and hurting because of it. It was only after I decided to give God my body as well as my soul and spirit, and after I dedicated myself to the program I'm sharing with you, that I truly changed.

". . . Not by might, nor by power, but by my spirit, saith the Lord of hosts" (Zechariah 4:6) is true and real for you and me as we get our bodies into shape for the Master's use.

Your born-again body wants to be blessed. Your life was meant to be lived abundantly. What is it you would like the Lord to help you accomplish? Check below:

- ___✓___ more energy
- ___✓___ a happier disposition
- ___✓___ a thinner, trimmer body
- ___✓___ greater stamina
- ___✓___ healthier skin
- ___✓___ permanent weight loss
- ___✓___ muscle tone
- ___✓___ vibrant appearance
- ___✓___ new strength for the rest of your life

You can tell by the points you checked above that your body needs some loving attention. You are in charge of your body. Nobody else is. You can stop pinning the blame for your flabby midriff on your job. You can bless your midriff and your knees and calves and feet, too, for that matter, by learning how to be in control of what your body looks like and the energy you have. No excuses, now.

Famous Excuses and the Wrong Solutions

Recognize any of these excuses for staying fat and out of shape?

Excuse	Solution
I'm nervous	Eat something
I'm worried	Eat some more
I'm angry	Go to dinner
I'm anxious	Snack after dinner
I'm lonely	Eat enough for two
I'm fearful	Take your cookies to bed with you

I'm not trying to pry, but haven't you excused your chubbiness and out-of-shapeness on things like loneliness? Carolyn M. once spent the entire evening sitting at her kitchen counter, eating cheese and crackers and drinking diet soda while telling herself that nobody would ever love her because she was too fat.

I know about loneliness, too. I've spent more days and nights and months and years walking alone, watching happy couples walk hand in hand, than I can stand. Don't tell me about loneliness. Single people know. As a speaker, I do a lot of traveling each year. Alone. I know all about cold and friendless airports, hotels, train stations; strange countries and faces; long hours with no one to talk to.

Once in Vienna, I had walked the streets for several hours before finally deciding to stop to eat. I had spent the afternoon in Sigmund Freud's personal library doing some research, and I wanted to walk and go out for dinner. I was stunned when I saw I was the only single woman in the restaurant. Now I ask you, what was I to do? What would *you* have done?

1. Pulled out your Bible, stood on the table, and taken the opportunity to preach in German?
2. Cowered in a corner and hoped the host would seat you where nobody would point and laugh at you, or worse, try to pick you up?
3. Rushed out and gone to the nearest grocer for a log of strudel, some sandwiches, and soda to eat alone in your hotel room?

I'm pleased to tell you I did none of the above, but pulled myself erect, prayed for courage, and enjoyed a light, happy, and quite "alone" meal. I felt in control that day. A stressful situation is something we all try to avoid. Handling stress, facing it and not running away from it, gives us a sense of dignity and strength.

Nobody likes to be lonely. When you feel lonely, self-pity becomes a roaring giant within you. You make choices that may be destructive. Overeating, not exercising, running away from life, or choosing situations that will abuse your integrity are not God's design for you. Since I have wrestled with overeating most of my life, I find that it is something I will be tempted to do whenever I allow self-pity to pay a call. Remember, self-pity can try to visit, but you don't have to open the door and let it in.

Call it any name you will, an excuse is an *excuse*. The reason we get out of shape is that we make excuses not to exercise, like:

- I'm too busy.
- I'm sick.
- I can't afford the sneakers. (Then borrow some.)
- There's not enough room. (Make

room. After you're in shape, you will move the furniture in half the time.)
- I don't want to ruin my hair and nails. (Don't let them ruin you.)
- I'm in Vienna.
- My husband likes me the way I am. (You want to bet?)
- I need the extra weight to keep me warm in the winter. (I've never seen a fat person without a winter coat, same as thin persons.)
- I don't want to get muscular like those lady wrestlers.
- Exercise is tiresome. (Flab is more tiresome.)

Before beginning this program, please pray with me right now, realizing that all things are possible in Christ Jesus.

Dear Lord, I give You my body so that You can teach me how to take care of it. I choose to be physically fit and strong for Your sake. I refuse pride and the ways of vanity and self-vaunting in order to be fully dedicated to You. I commit myself to You in every area of my life—body, soul, and spirit—in Jesus' name. Amen.

If you prayed that prayer with me, you are ready to begin. The Lord loves *all* of you. He wants you to be healthy and complete in every aspect of life. Perhaps physical fitness has been a horrendous lack in your life, making you a pawn for sickness, emotional disturbances, lethargy, and a varied array of problems. I am not offering you false promises when I promise that the Lord is faithful and will be faithful to you as you start this program and continue it with Him. You will experience an incredible emotional and physical boost almost immediately.

In preparing this book I took an aerobics class every single day along with my own regular Blessercize program. I also ran five days a week, working up to my present rate of thirty miles a week. Now, at my counseling and fitness center in San Diego, we have Blessercize classes all day long, as well as a total fitness program. The difference between our attitudes and the attitudes of the non-Christian groups are remarkable. Instead of moaning and groaning or complaining about sore muscles, our Fun to Be Fit people exult, "I'm making my body happy!"

You can make your body happy, too.

Because you care and will soon realize how much the Lord cares, you will give your body the attention it has been begging for. I believe in you because I know the Lord does. He says we can do all things through Christ who strengthens us. Praise God! Let's get strong together for God now.

2

Getting on Speaking Terms With Your Body

When was the last time you had a good conversation with your body? Usually people talk *about* their bodies, but rarely *to* them. "Oh, I hate my feet," someone will say, or, "My arms are too short," or too long, or, "I'm too fat," skinny, whatever.

Keeping this book in your hand, I want you to find a mirror and take a good look at yourself. Now say, "Hello, [*your name*]. Hello, [*your name*]'s body. I bless you in the name of Jesus."

Tell your body you're going to begin exercising it to *really* bless yourself.

A survey made for the President's Council on Physical Fitness and Sports showed that 55 percent of the nation's adults engage in some sort of exercise. When the activities themselves were analyzed, though, it became apparent that at least 80 percent of the people were not exercising sufficiently or properly to avoid physiological breakdown. Exercise, as we are accustomed to it, is not only boring and ineffective but dangerous as well. Calisthenics, for example, originated in Sweden where the landowners drilled the peasants to bear themselves like soldiers with calisthenic drills using militaristic, precise, geometric movements that were unnatural and difficult. Chest up, shoulders back, head erect, and a straight, flat back is pain producing. Modern exercise programs are often so rigorous that injuries result. When I was a ballet dancer, I can safely say that every person in our ballet company had suffered some sort of injury through dancing. When I studied at the Metropolitan Opera School of the Ballet in New York City, as well as with the most famous jazz dance teachers in the country, not one professional dancer I knew did not suffer some sort of malady because of our painful and strenuous workouts and routines.

The current fitness rage and the fitness cults which have emerged in recent years seem to stress that good physical condition depends upon exhaustion and painful, strenuous workouts. The program you are about to begin is aerobic as well as anaerobic. You will exercise your heart as well as your muscles. Your body will get a total workout every day, *without* torture. Exercise is so often thought of as two extremes. At one end of the spectrum are the Olympic stars, and at the other end are people who do almost no exercise at all. We hire athletes to perform for us, and we buy energy-saving equipment to keep us from exercising. Exercise, however, means to prolong our lives and to add vitality to everything we do. Inactivity will do us in.

Without proper exercise, we are more likely to suffer from such maladies as hypertension, lower-back problems, heart problems, excess weight, chronic fatigue, and even emotional disorders such as depression. Almost everybody wants to be strong and healthy but we do little, or the wrong things, to get that way. It's been said that the typical job in a modern office requires less physical exertion than taking a shower.

Your body is designed to be used, and it can actually be used vigorously without breaking into bits, like glass. The secret is knowing *how* to use your body. The damage you do to your body can be due to *not* exercising as well as how you do exercise. Your muscles are the lifeguards of your body. Your muscle structure must be strong and toned in order to support your skeletal structure and to protect your spine.

Doctors recommend exercise for such physical problems as varicose veins, arthritis, migraine headaches, menstrual cramps, and even nicotine and alcohol cravings. Exercise will decrease the level of cholesterol in your blood and produce chemicals in the body that act as natural antidepressants. I'll bet you weren't even aware of what you've been missing all this time.

Your Metabolism

There's more. Exercise affects your metabolism, which is the combustion process that goes on in your cells when carbohydrates in the form of glucose or glycogen and oxygen are burned, creating energy. The energy released as all this is going on is measured in calories. That's why we say we "burn up calories." Your metabolic rate goes up when you exercise vigorously, and it takes more time to slow down again afterward. This means you actually continue to burn calories even after you stop exercising. The greater the ratio of lean tissue you have to body fat, the more calories you will burn. This is because lean tissue is more highly oxygenated than fat, and it keeps the metabolic process going longer. If you exercise long enough at one time, your muscles use fat for fuel instead of carbohydrates. Your endurance is increased because your muscles will program to store the carbohydrates instead of the fat.

You can throw away that old excuse about having a very slow metabolism, and you can stop saying that everything you eat turns to fat. Your metabolism is a process of breaking down the food you eat. If you stopped eating such heavy, fattening foods, your metabolism would be a lot happier.

Your Know You're Out of Shape When . . .

- Your friends plan a short bike trip and invite your bike to go but not you.
- The last time you rode your bicycle was in junior high school.

- You wait twenty minutes for an elevator rather than walk up four flights of stairs.
- You don't get a dog because walking it each day would take too much energy.
- All your hobbies take place at the dinner table or in the kitchen.
- You're the only one at a party who thinks jumping rope is detrimental to human health.
- Your legs hurt each time you get up to change the channel on the TV.
- Your favorite part of a television exercise show is the cooking segment.
- You choose Miss Piggy as "Athlete of the Year."
- Your children buy you leotards and tights for Christmas instead of the ice-cream maker you asked for.
- You think the word *aerobics* has something to do with jet travel.
- Your eighty-some-year-old Great-Uncle Fred can do sit-ups faster than you.
- You're the only one who doesn't wear a jogging suit to bridge club.
- You're the only one at the office who'd rather eat than play volleyball at lunchtime.
- Your husband stops insisting you're not fat, just sensual—and starts using the word *portly* with frequency.
- You tell others with firm conviction that manufacturers are making clothes much smaller nowadays.

Stress and Exercise

Caroline R. is a healthy-looking, twenty-one-year-old college senior. Her busy schedule includes working part-time as a waitress at a local restaurant, teaching private piano lessons on Saturday, leading the junior choir at church, and occasionally jogging if there is someone to jog with. Approximately once a week she plays tennis with her boyfriend.

"I'm always tired, Marie," she tells me over the telephone. "I'm going to have to drop something from my schedule, but I don't know which activity should go."

Caroline made an appointment to see me, and we surveyed her situation.

"Maybe it's not dropping something you should consider," I suggested. "Perhaps what you need is to *add* something to your schedule."

Caroline was surprised at such a notion. "Are you kidding? I couldn't add one more thing to this life of mine. I'm already practically on the verge of a nervous breakdown."

Caroline's case is somewhat typical of many of us. Her healthy appearance is deceiving. (No, being thin does *not* mean you're healthy!) Caroline was caught in a web of being depressed and tired, so she ate less healthy foods, exercised less, and felt worse and worse.

> Being tired + overwork + poor nutrition + lack of exercise = tiredness, depression, and lack of energy.

Caroline complained of frequent colds and headaches along with a variety of other physical symptoms, including menstrual cramps, irritability, and constipation. I suggested a program of regular daily exercise to get herself into shape so she could handle the demands of her life. She also needed to change her diet to feed her body the foods it craved in order to bless herself.

"Martin Luther was a busy man, too, Caroline," I told her. "He didn't cut things out of his schedule when he needed more strength. Instead he added more. On one particularly busy day he was known to have said, 'The day ahead of me is so demanding and so busy that I must begin it with at least three hours of prayer.' "

Caroline was a victim of stress, that's true, but there's nobody who can get out of this life without ever having experienced stress. God has given us sure-fire ways of handling these stresses of life. The three culprits robbing Caroline of health and vitality were *lack of prayer, proper diet,* and *physical exercise.*

If your body is under emotional and physical stress, it will release the hormone adrenaline. Without regular exercise, the adrenaline tends to accumulate in your body until it reaches a danger point. Too much adrenaline can flood your system and give you a sense of fatigue and irritability. If you engage in a daily exercise program, you'll increase your metabolism, which uses up the excess adrenaline. Instead of being emotionally tense and nervous, you should be energized.

When I taught Speech and Communication in a Bible college in Minnesota, I was aware of the emotional stress on the students on the days they were to give their speeches. Some of them were actually sick with fear, no matter how hard they prayed.

I taught Exercises to Relax By along with the regular course work. On the days of their speeches, I instructed the students to exercise before class. Just a short warm-up, mind you, to be done in the bathroom or anyplace there might be privacy. Some deep breathing, knee bends, touching of the toes, arm swings, head rolls, and they were sufficiently loosened up to face what lay ahead. The exercises helped and the students arrived in class less tense and in better control.

If you're blaming your middle-age spread on the fact that you lead a life of stress, you can drop that excuse right now. You still must live with your own hips and your own stomach, no matter

how stressful your life is. You can't tell me that only fat people have stress. The next time you reach for the cupboard door for a little something when you're under pressure, slap your hand and say, "Eating is not a reward for the energy I spend being distressed or under stress."

Facts to Tell Your Body

- Muscle weighs more than fat and takes up less space, so you will lose inches as well as pounds on your Fun to Be Fit program, though at times it may seem your scale is not your friend. If you exercise every day, you may find that you weigh more than someone who is fatter than you, although you're a size 4 and they're a size 13. It's your muscles. Praise the Lord for your muscles and bless them. They weigh more than fat.

- The most fattening thing in your life is self-pity, not rich food.

- It is not true that females are more prone to injury during physical activity than males. In fact, we have a subcutaneous layer of fat as an extra cushion to protect us. Self-neglect is what makes you vulnerable to injury.

- Only 3 percent of the population suffers from thyroid problems. Your hormones and glands can be taught to behave themselves with help from your doctor or endocrinologist, and a little help from *you.* (Like stop telling yourself you're fat and out of shape because of a thyroid problem that doesn't exist.)

- Talking on the telephone uses fifty calories an hour, so just by calling your mother you can use up those four cashews you sneaked at lunch.

- Nancy Reagan eats her vegetables plain, too, so enjoy.

- Due to a shortage of testosterone in the female system, women are generally not capable of developing large, defined muscle groups. So don't worry about looking like a candidate for Muscle Beach. You're not going to get bulging, knotty muscles on this program.
- Your body only requires one gram of salt a day (a fifth of a teaspoon) in order to keep a good balance going.
- Diet soda is high in sodium and will assist your tissues in retaining fluid, and actually hinder the weight loss process in your body. These diet sodas are chemical laden and unhealthy; if you really want to bless your body, drink fresh fruit juices and beautiful, exciting *water*.
- Research has shown that what you eat early in the day is less fattening than what you eat at night because at night the food you eat is absorbed into your bloodstream more slowly. When you exercise, your blood sugar level remains stable because your muscles use more fat than sugar proportionately as fuel, and there is less insulin in your blood. It's when your blood sugar drops that you feel hungry. What I'm telling you is, eat a big breakfast, a small dinner, exercise with me on this new program, and you'll bless your body like never before.
- One ounce of ricotta cheese contains forty-two calories. (Well, that's better than peanut butter, which has one hundred calories a tablespoon, isn't it? I'm only trying to look on the bright side of things.)
- Once on the program, you will discover you can accomplish a lot more during the day with much less fatigue. This is because when your muscle tissue is stimulated, it gains in endurance.
- After being on your new program for three to six months, you can expect your body to more effectively resist illnesses such as colds and flus because of your more efficient body system. You can also expect to be less prone to injury, because your body will be more flexible, surefooted, and strong.

Doesn't that sound wonderful?
What are we waiting for?

3

Reaching Your Full Potential in Body, Soul, and Spirit

A Total Picture

A young woman I'll call Rodna came into my office, complaining of severe depression. She had a number of physiological complaints as well. Rodna told me nothing seemed to be going well in her life. She said she was a Christian and she attended church as regularly as she could, but she just didn't seem to feel God was on her side.

Upon first meeting Rodna, one would assume she had her life fairly together. She dressed well, had a happy expression on her face, and seemed to carry herself with a certain degree of confidence. After spending time with Rodna, however, these attributes gradually crumbled.

Once her facade was down, it was apparent that Rodna needed to know that love and acceptance are not things we need to earn. She was a woman of twenty-seven who had lived most of those years buying tickets to life. She viewed her world as a hostile one that had to be penetrated with hard work, effort, and Brownie points to win acceptance. Rodna began to read *Telling Yourself the Truth*, the book I coauthored with Dr. Bill Backus, and started applying the principles we outline in it.

"I know now that God wants me to reach my full potential," Rodna told me emotionally. "I just don't know how to get there."

Being fit physically molds into the total picture of your being. Rodna had already tried a number of things to straighten out her life. She had belonged to self-help groups, been to therapists, experienced a marriage and a divorce, and tried to comfort herself through drinking, drugs, and overeating. She now knew that all of her attempts at alleviating pain and finding happiness were in vain. Even though Rodna was a Christian, she had not come into a place of joy and peace as the preachers told her she would if she would just go to church faithfully, pray regularly, and read her Bible.

"What's wrong with me, Marie?" she begged, in a tone so pitiful it wrenched my heart.

Make an Agreement With Yourself

Before we can be the persons God intended us to be, we have to make an agreement with ourselves regarding the source of our strength. As a therapist and teacher, I often think of the words of the Apostle Paul in Galatians 4:19, when he was writing to the churches throughout Galatia: "My little children, of whom I travail in birth again *until Christ be formed in you*" (my italics). Paul had travailed in birth for these people, but Christ had not been formed in them. It is Christ Himself who desires full access to our spirits, souls, and bodies so that He can be completed in us, and we in Him.

For no man can lay a foundation other than the one which is laid, which is Jesus Christ. Now if any man builds upon the foundation with gold, silver, precious stones, wood, hay, straw, each man's work will become evident; for the day will show it, because it is to be revealed with fire; and the fire itself will test the quality of each man's work. If any man's work which he has built upon it remains, he shall receive a reward. If any man's work is burned up, he shall suffer loss; but he himself shall be saved, yet so as through fire. Do you not know that you are a temple of God, and that the Spirit of God dwells in you? If any man destroys the temple of God, God will destroy him, for the temple of God is holy, and that is what you are.

1 Corinthians 3:11–17 NASB

There's no person born, yesterday, today, or ever, who is able to live to his full potential without God. Rodna knew that, and maybe you do, too. Your human weaknesses tell you. Jesus told us that when we are weak, we can be strong, because in our weaknesses *God* is made strong in us.

Many people have developed strong human abilities, and inner strength to get them through life with great success and skill. Don't be deceived. They are not living up to their full potential if God is not at the core of their being. Verse 18 (NASB) follows:

Let no man deceive himself. If any man among you thinks that he is wise in this age, let him become foolish that he may become wise.

Rodna thought she was a failure in life because A) she told herself she was, and B) when she looked around she thought others were more successful and happy than she was.

The reason she believed these things, which were essentially misbeliefs, was that she did not realize no one on earth was more unique or special than she. She had never faced head-on these words of God: "I have called thee with an everlasting love: therefore with loving-kindness have I drawn thee" (Jeremiah 31:3). She believed other people were more loved than she and certainly more deserving of love. Because of this, she worked overtime for acceptance from others. When she got it, she worried that she wouldn't keep it. Also, it was such hard work to be accepted that it was hardly worth the agony.

How could Rodna reach her full potential in body, soul, and spirit, when her human weaknesses were being mistaken for the foundation of her life? Her foundation was Jesus Christ, and He is not weak!

When we build our lives on wood, hay, and stubble, what should we expect when a lighted match is set to it? Naturally our own human strength will fail. Even if it looks as though those non-Christians around the corner are pillars of power and might, God tells us plainly, "Let no man glory in men" (1 Corinthians 3:21), and goes on to say: *"For all things are your's!"* (my italics).

Rodna began to examine her life with new eyes. In addition to her regular therapy sessions with me, she came to our Blessercize classes three times a week, and also started a regular running program. Today, Rodna is twenty-two pounds lighter, in shape, and holding down a demanding executive position in the company where she works. Hers is a happy ending, not only because she learned how to teach herself to be happy and learned how to tell herself the truth but also because she learned she *could* reach her full potential as a Christian person. Rodna's life is really just beginning now because depression no longer plagues her. Her circumstances have changed because *she* changed them. She took hold of the reins of heaven by the power of the Holy Spirit, and chose to see herself as God saw her. Rodna stuck to her program faithfully and, in fact, when I had to cancel an appointment once because I was out of town speaking, she was deeply distressed. For a person who had once been unable to show up anywhere on time, and one who habitually broke engagements and appointments, her new behavior was nothing short of incredible.

Rodna told me just last week something I'll never forget. I want them to be your words, too: "I feel for the first time in my life I'm really *me*, and you know what? Me is beautiful!"

Your Potential Means Following a Schedule

One of the reasons Rodna's story has a happy ending is that she followed a schedule. She learned how to discipline herself, even when she didn't feel like it. Think of your favorite heroes and heroines in history for a moment. What is the secret of a great man or woman? I think we could answer that in two words: self-control and perseverence. I can't imagine Joan of Arc, leading ten thousand troops to war, pausing in the middle of battle at Orleans to sigh wistfully, "What I wouldn't give for a plate of french fries."

If You Are Drop-out Prone

If you are drop-out prone, I want to give you some strategies designed to help you stay on your program. They are effective if you will commit yourself to following them.

1. *Have a convenient place to exercise.* Rod Dishman, Ph.D., sports psychologist and professor in the department of Health and Physical Education at Southwest Missouri State University in Springfield, says business executives are much more likely to be active in an exercise program if they have easy access to an exercise facility. Finnish researchers and a study conducted at the University of Wisconsin show that college professors who chose to get involved in an exercise program and were still involved seven years later were closer to an exercise area than professors who were not involved in exercising. You do not have to be a business executive or a professor to have your exercise area near you. But be sure your exercise area is close enough and easy enough to get to so that it is not discouraging. I know one lady who set

up a section of her garage to exercise in, but she doesn't use it often. The last time I talked with her she told me she hadn't exercised in over a month. Upon visiting her and taking a peek at her exercise area in the garage, it was not hard to understand why she stayed away. The garage was cold and dark, and her exercise area was difficult to reach because of the car, bicycles, and other paraphernalia in the way. I suggested she set up an exercise area in her dining room just by moving a few chairs back each day. She did this, and it is working out very well.

2. *Make your goals long-range.* If you haven't exercised for many years, you may not look like an Olympic gymnast after your first two weeks of the program. Dramatic changes will not occur overnight, although they will occur eventually. If you plan to look terrific and fit by next summer instead of next week, you will not be so discouraged, nor will you be so hard on yourself. Don't compete. God has shown us, "If any man's work abide which he hath built thereupon, he shall receive a reward" (1 Corinthians 3:14). You know that you *will* reap the reward of your labors if you remain faithful.

3. *Understand your body.* Not everyone has the ability to become a professional athlete, but everyone can improve his or her physical condition. Knowing your body will help you to know how far you can expect yourself to go. Your most important goal should be to be healthy and fit physically, mentally, emotionally, and spiritually.

4. *Pain is not always a virtue.* Your heart rate, muscular pain, body temperature, and breathing all tell you whether you're working too strenuously or not. If you are putting too much metabolic stress on your cardiovascular system, slow down. When you are running or engaged in any aerobic activity, your rule of thumb is that you ought to be able to carry on a comfortable conversation without gagging, gasping, choking, wheezing, or struggling.

5. *Be sure to keep a daily exercise log.* Drop-out prone personalities usually feel discouraged when there is slow improvement. Keeping a log will buoy up your spirits. This log will reinforce you and serve as a reward because you can see how much work you're putting into your physical fitness program, and be proud of yourself. "Well done, good and faithful servant" (*see* Matthew 25:21) should ring in your ears.

6. *Keep the fun in your fitness program.* When I first began jogging a few years ago, my efforts were usually in spurts. I worked so hard at improving my time and increasing my mileage that the fun just wore out. I started to avoid my daily jogging time and gradually I would stop altogether, only to try again a couple of weeks or months later. When exercise is no longer fun, it becomes drudgery. You feel you're competing with some invisible force, some fitness monster who thrives on sadistic demands. Sometimes you may not feel like running as far and as intensely as you did yesterday. Don't push yourself. Enjoy yourself. Your body loves you, and you don't have to worry that it will scold you for not improving your time or breaking any records. You are not competing with anyone. Keeping on the program is what is important. Exercising your heart and burning calories are important, but your goal is simply to stick on the program, no matter what. If your best friend can do eighty sit-ups and you're still doing ten, just praise the Lord, because last year at this time you weren't doing any.

7. *Involve somebody else.* Some people love to run with a companion, and exercise in a group. Aerobic exercises like tennis, racquetball, ice skating, and roller skating can be done with others. Bicycling, jumping rope, and rebound jumping can also be done with others. Fitness can bring a family together like you can't imagine. I have mothers and daughters in my Blessercize classes and whole families joining in aerobics activities. Surprisingly, only about 50 percent of

the population is involved in some form of physical activity, and 50 percent of these people drop out within six months. But not you. You can be very proud of yourself for maintaining your fitness program. Yours is a lifetime thing. You will bless not only yourself but your family and many others as well.

By this is My Father glorified, that you bear much fruit, and so prove to be My disciples.

John 15:8 NASB

And whatever we ask we receive from Him, because we keep His commandments and do the things that are pleasing in His sight.

1 John 3:22 NASB

4

Beyond Yourself

How Persevering Are You?

Grade: 3/26

To rate yourself on how persevering you are, read each of the following statements and write after each item your answer—"Often," "Sometimes," or "Never"—to describe how characteristic the statement is when applied to you.

Grade:

3 1. I'm good at keeping promises, especially the ones I make to myself. ___O___

3 2. I'm good at making decisions and standing by them. ___O

2 3. I do not avoid stressful situations. ___S

3 4. I feel my well-being is my own responsibility and not someone else's. ___O

3 5. My activities are planned and well scheduled. ___O

2 6. I can handle stressful situations, even though I'd rather avoid them. ___S

2 7. I do not quit a task even though I feel tired. ___S

3 8. I like to set goals and work toward accomplishing them. ___O

2 9. I'm a self-starter and rarely need to be pushed to get things done. ___S

3/26 10. I always meet deadlines and I can be depended upon to get things done that have to be done. ___O___

Scoring yourself: Give yourself three points for each "Often." "Sometimes" gives you two points, and "Never" will earn you one point. Add up your score.

30–24: <u>You're achievement prone.</u> Chances are, you are a person who is busier than most people and yet always has time for people who are in need or to do something good for yourself. You are not only a person of intense motivation but you also have the ability to persevere. Be easy on yourself because you may have a tendency to drive yourself a little too hard. You will do very well on your Fun to Be Fit program. Slow and easy should be your motto.

24–18: You are motivated and are actually within the average range of stick-to-itness. You will do very well on this program because chances are, you're tired of being lazy. Your self-image is healthy, and it will improve as you go along.

18–12: Your level of achievement depends upon your moods and feelings. Relationships may come first in your life, even before your own wants and interests. In the past you would exercise only if a friend joined you. My Rx: Read *Telling Yourself the Truth* twice.

12 and under: Come on, now. You may not have had much self-discipline in the past, but that's no reason for you to stay that way. Almost everybody, at some time or another in their lives, must face change. I'm on your side and you're going to make it. Chin up—it may be hard at first, but with God as the strength of your life, you cannot fail. For you to fail means God has to fail, and that's impossible.

The strategies I've given you will help you to understand yourself and get through the first critical weeks of this program. I cannot stress enough how important the first weeks are. They will set the momentum for you, and you will begin to feel the exhilaration of fitness. It is that feeling and that joy which is something so indescribably sublime that I want it for you more than anything. You are not going to be one of those people who say, "I tried but I couldn't stay with it," because you are filled with the power of the Spirit of God, and it is He who is strengthening you as you obey Him.

Reaching Beyond Yourself

When I stood in the rooms of Mozart's house in Vienna, Austria, on Domgasse a while back, I shuddered with awe.

Mozart's musical genius brought him no great wealth; it didn't even secure his health. His *Requiem Mass* is recognized as one of the most powerful pieces of music ever written. I stood in the room where he composed it and remembered the electrifying beauty of the music. Even as Mozart lay dying in that room, he was silently singing the notes of the Judgment Day trumpet in *Requiem*. How I love that piece of music. Mozart died at thirty-six after completing it. He heard the music of heaven and gave it to us through his suffering. I know people who go to pieces when they get a common cold, and they can do nothing but watch TV and eat. They're debilitated. Not Mozart. I just can't see him sniveling away and lamenting, "If only I'd taken up business administration." He reached beyond his own strength. (I can't help but wonder how much more he could have done if he had been physically fit!)

I think of Daniel of the Bible, who rose from utter desolation to a position of great prominence. I look at his life and I'm inspired to know the Lord as he did. God is no respecter of persons, and offers the same strength of character to you and me that He offered to your favorite heroes, if indeed they are heroes. I want you to see yourself as a *strong* person, a person of integrity. You're going to be a person who is physically fit as well as spiritually fit. Treat yourself with respect.

Why This Program Is Different From Any Other Fitness Program You've Tried Before

It is the *inner* person we are really developing here. Your outside will show it, but your inner person is the one who really benefits.

That he would grant you, according to the riches of his glory, to be strengthened with might by his Spirit in the inner man.

Ephesians 3:16

When we read the words "grieve not the Holy Spirit of God, whereby ye are sealed unto the day of redemption" (Ephesians 4:30), we cannot neglect to realize our bodies, which are the temple of the Holy Spirit. How awful for Him not to be able to get into and fully use His own temple! Maybe He has your heart, your thoughts, your good deeds, but your poor body is in sad shape. The temple of the Holy Spirit is property condemned, uninhabitable, weak at every seam.

Now I'm not trying to upset you, but I do want you to see that *Fun to Be Fit* is a spiritual endeavor as well as a physical one. The Bible also tells us in 1 Timothy 4:8 to exercise ourselves unto godliness:

For bodily exercise profiteth little: but godliness is profitable unto all things. . . .

We are training ourselves toward godliness in order to please God. This we do in *every area of our lives.*

Becoming Strong

Your goal is to be strong *inside* in order to shine outside. Your body is about to become stronger, healthier, and more attractive. The Lord knew what He was talking about when He spoke through Timothy to tell us physical exercise is a waste of time. Of course it is a waste of time if it is without *Him.* You can join all the spas and exercise groups you want, lose weight, get in shape, but believe me, if the Lord Jesus isn't Lord over your labors, the most you will gain is pride. I have seen people topple right out of the arms of God because their fitness programs were executed in vanity. They used sexy, lustful music to work out to, they talked body talk only, spent long hours in front of the spa mirrors, watched their bodies tone and firm up, and what happened? Their clothes became sexier, their walks a little more haughty, their choices a little more liberal, and *zappo,* right into the clutches

of the devil they fell. Sin overtook them. Nothing could be more tragic.

Jesus said to *resist the devil,* not join him.

Pride is a killer. It's the devil's biggest weapon against you. He wants you to become physically oriented in order to keep your mind off God. I want you to decide right now before turning another page of this book that you are going to engage in this program because you want to experience God more fully.

You'll never have the body the Lord wants you to have without having His mind as well. "Let this mind be in you, which was also in Christ Jesus," the Apostle Paul wrote (Philippians 2:5). The Lord Jesus was humble, obedient, and took upon Himself the form of a servant.

I'm not going to ask you to look in a mirror before you begin the program, to identify your bulges, problem areas, and weaknesses. I will, however, ask you to search your heart for a moment—your spiritual heart. Have you ever given God the right to your physical health? Have you ever dedicated yourself to Him as a healthy, *fit* person?

In the hundreds of services and meetings I have spoken at across the United States and in other countries, I always pray for the sick. When people come forward at the end of the meeting, no matter where I am, at least half of the people ask for prayer for physical healing. Because I am a psychotherapist, I also receive requests for prayer for emotional and mental healing, but usually most of the requests are for physical healing. Why is this?

On one end of our spectrum there is the sickly and neglected body and on the other, the proud, athletic one. Often we spend more time praying for our bodies when we are sick than when we are well. We need to learn how to *bless* our bodies so that the Lord is always the Master and Guardian of our total selves.

You need to know how to bless yourself before you can truly bless someone else. Your body is, sadly enough, the most neglected part of you. You don't have to be a victim of sickness, weakness, lethargy, depression, sloth, lackluster, overweight, or tiredness anymore! You also can be free of vanity and pride. Being out of shape and staying that way can be a form of pride. *You* can decide now to bless yourself. You can decide to change. Your mind was given to you so that you could use it to make godly choices for yourself and your world. Use it now to choose God's plan for health and fitness.

I want you to be able to say to me:

Yes, Marie, I choose to dedicate myself to being physically fit as well as spiritually fit.

I choose to reach my full potential as the person God created me to be. I choose to give the Lord my body so the Holy Spirit can live in a clean, health temple and so I can live my life glorifying Him as a healthier, happier person. I choose to love and bless my body.

Okay, this is serious now. I want you to commit yourself to your promise by signing your name to it.

Yes, Marie, I'm ready to begin my Fun to Be Fit program. I will exercise myself unto godliness and glorify God with my body, soul, and spirit.

_____

(Your Name)

_____

11/4/90

(Date)

5

Living in Your Body

The Joy of Sweat

The first time Claire T. actually perspired during a workout, she got so excited she called her mother. "Guess what, Mom!"

"Don't tell me. You're calling collect?"

"Good heavens, Mom. This is *spiritual.*"

"You're calling collect from China?"

"Mother, listen—you'll never believe it—I'm—well, I'm *sweating!*"

"You're—?"

"It's wonderful! I haven't sweated in years! I actually exercised until I sweat. Isn't it exciting?"

"You called me long-distance, collect, to tell me you're *sweating?*"

"But don't you see, Mom? I'm getting *fit.* I just know it. God is going to bless me. I've never been able to stick with exercising before until I actually sweat!"

Claire's enthusiasm can only be understood if you know what it's like to feel your body suddenly come alive after living in a veritable bowl of Jell-O for so many years. Claire was a person who wasn't really fat—she was "pleasantly plump" and totally out of shape. The only time she ever perspired was if she was somehow caught in the summertime where there was no air conditioning. Physical exertion had no place in her life.

You should see Claire today—fit, happy, trim, and very grateful to the Lord for helping her find her potential.

"I owe it all to sweat," she proudly told my beginners' aerobics class.

It's *good* for you to sweat. Don't knock it until you've tried it, as they say. The exercises you are going to do in this program will require your dedication at least thirty minutes three times a week. (At *least,* I said.) The exercises are carefully planned to use each part of your body in a sequence. The most effective workout is when you vigorously sustain the use of your entire body for at least thirty minutes. You will work up to this time, beginning slowly. If you are in terrible shape, you can begin with five- to fifteen-minute workouts, gradually working up to thirty minutes each exercise period.

Vigorous exercise is necessary to tone your muscles, burn calories, improve your circulation, eliminate toxins, and strengthen your heart and lungs. It's a myth that a few push-ups before bed will benefit your body to any great degree. Of course, I'm all for a few push-ups over none at all, but I want you to discard the old notion that physical exercise is some sort of option to you.

Discard the idea that if you do ten knee bends and ten sit-ups upon arising, that's all you need. You're only fooling yourself. These little "token" body movements do no good whatsoever for your cardiovascular system, or anything else, for that matter.

Steve, a forty-four-year-old business executive, is a typical case in point. He told me about his daily exercise regimen of a five-minute token workout before going to bed each night. "Not enough to make you sweat," I commented. He agreed. Never once had his knee bends and stretches produced a drop of sweat. He would have done just as well strolling the patio. I questioned him about his physical activity during the rest of his ordinary day. I learned he spent his time either in the car or at a desk, still sitting, riding, or standing. The most exercise he engaged in was walking from his office to a restaurant a block away for lunch. Steve's major complaint was weakness and lack of energy. He was worried that there was something physically wrong with him. "Must be old age setting in," he conceded. (If there's one statement I hate, it's that one. Tell me you're getting old and my toes automatically curl under.)

In exactly one month's time, Steve's physical and emotional states radically changed. I developed a daily jogging program for him with warm-up and cool-down exercises, and supplemented it with working out with weights three times a week. The results were excellent. He not only lost weight but he also felt great.

I asked Steve what he thought made the biggest difference in his program. He said, "Working at it. Instead of playing at exercises or avoiding them altogether, I am now working at a definite program. I'm working up a *sweat*." (There's that word *sweat* again.)

Your exercise program is a total body, soul, and spirit approach. Like Steve, you will begin each exercise session with a warm-up. Gradually you work muscles, strengthening and conditioning, before beginning the aerobic part of your session. You will work up to your natural pace, to a sweat, and then finish with your cool-down exercises.

There are approximately 639 muscles and 208 bones in your body. Just think how happy they'll be now that you're going to give them some attention. After all, they deserve a little fun in life, too.

Your Blood and How It Works

Your body has sixty thousand miles of blood vessels (seventy-five thousand if you're a man). This life flow within you carries oxygen, water, nutrients, hormones, protective antibodies, and dozens of other vital substances to each of your 60 trillion cells. Your blood repairs biological damage, gets rid of cellular waste, and works overtime when you're sick.

Cholesterol, the Life Robber

When your doctor tells you he's going to take some blood tests to test your blood chemistry, one of the things you will be tested for is cholesterol. This is a fatty substance found in the blood. It clogs up your arteries and contributes to the cause of heart attacks and strokes. At least 1 million Americans die each year from heart and blood vessel disorders. Inactivity is a contributor to this killer disease.

A high level of cholesterol contributes to the formation of fatty plaques along the inside wall of the blood vessels. As the fatty particles build up, a layer at a time, the inner diameter of the vessel becomes smaller, slowing the rate of blood flow and making the heart work harder to force the blood through the restricted orifice. Dr. Kenneth Cooper, the father of aerobics, found that aerobic exercise lowers the cholesterol risk by altering the cholesterol form as it appears in the bloodstream. Endocrinologists say exercise could prevent fatty particles from building up.

The main source of cholesterol is meat. Beef, pork, lamb, chicken, and turkey contain between 75 and 125 milligrams of cholesterol per serving. Dairy products and eggs are also high in cholesterol. An overabundance of cholesterol in the system can cause hardening of the arteries (arteriosclerosis) as well as gallstones. Boo to cholesterol!

Oxygen

The key to a healthy heart, lungs, and cardiovascular system is oxygen. The body can store food but it can't store oxygen. The body uses the food it wants and stores the rest, but not so with oxygen. Oxygen has to be constantly replenished in our bodies. The blood needs oxygen. When you exercise, you are pumping more blood and increasing the efficiency of your heart. You increase the number and size of the blood vessels that carry the blood to your body tissue, saturating the tissues throughout your whole body with energy-producing oxygen. Exercise will increase your total blood volume and improve the tone of your blood vessels, often reducing blood pressure in the process. In other words, you can win your war with cholesterol with your new exercise program.

Your Blood Pressure and Pulse

Your blood pressure and pulse are two of the most important indicators of the condition of your circulatory system. That's why the doctor checks these things first. Every time your heart contracts or beats, it pushes your blood out to all points of your body. When you place your fingertips lightly on your pulse points, you can feel your pulse as your blood moves through your arteries with each contraction. The slower the pulse rate, the more efficiently your heart is beating. In other words, your heart is sending out more blood with fewer contractions per minute. The average person's heart beats about seventy times a minute when at rest. There are some super athletes with much lower resting pulse rates. Björn Borg's, for instance, is said to be only thirty-six!

Blood pressure is the force that your blood applies against the walls of the vessels as it flows merrily through. It is recorded as two numbers, one written over the other. For example: 120/80. The top or systolic number is the pressure occurring in the blood vessels when your heart contracts. The bottom or diastolic number is the minimum pressure in the vessels as your heart rests between contractions.

You ought to know your blood pressure and have it checked about once a year. Most specialists agree that 120/80 is a good average pressure.

When you are out of condition, both your systolic and your diastolic figures are relatively higher, because your arteries tend to lose their elasticity and the resistance to blood flow increases. Certain factors can temporarily raise your normal blood pressure. James J. Lynch, Ph.D., professor of psychophysiology at the University of Maryland School of Medicine, discovered that even talking can lift blood pressure. He tested six hundred people of all ages, and almost without exception, blood pressure rose 10 to 50 percent when adults talked, babies cried, deaf people used sign language, and when people read aloud to themselves.

You have a problem with your blood pressure when it becomes high too often or stays up too long. If it bounces up and down like a yo-yo or takes too long to come down after being high, you could have a problem. Hypertension strikes 18 million American women a year and it is not only a disease of the elderly. Some other factors putting you at risk for high blood pressure are oral contraceptives, pregnancy, and menopause, according to cardiologist Harriet Dustean, M.D., formerly president of the American Heart Association. Don't panic if you have high blood pressure. Dr. Lewis Tobian, an expert on hypertensive therapy at the University of Minnesota Medical Center, says, "The combination of proper diet [lower in sodium and in calories for the overweight] and appropriate medication can lower the blood pressure to normal levels in virtually every hypertensive person."

At one time, the treatment of high blood pressure was rest and relaxation because it was associated with stress. Now, however, regular exercise has proven to be an effective means of neutralizing unavoidable daily stress. On your new exercise program, you are reducing the chances of cardiac failure because of the improved blood supply to your heart, which also keeps the surrounding heart tissue healthy. When fat circulates in your bloodstream for prolonged periods, the length of time it takes to get rid of it depends on your condition. If you are in good physical condition, it stands to reason that your body will get rid of the fat more quickly.

Take this moment to bless your blood system. I want you to speak to those trillions of blood cells now and tell them:

I bless my blood system now in the name of Jesus Christ. I bless my blood pressure, my blood chemistry, my blood count. Right now I bless the plasma, red cells, white cells, and platelets in my blood. I bring my entire vascular system under submission to the Word of God. The Word of God tells me it is the Spirit which gives life and therefore I now dedicate the blood pumping through this body to the Spirit of God to give life to.

But if the Spirit of him that raised up Jesus from the dead dwell in you, he that raised up Christ from the dead shall also quicken your mortal bodies by his Spirit that dwelleth in you.

Romans 8:11

Your Heart

That magnificent heart of yours, beautiful and marvelous, with its four-chambered muscular pump moving your six quarts of blood through your lungs and into your blood vessels, needs a great, big blessing from you. That sweet instrument of life in your body beats more than 36 million times a year. Now for all that work, don't you think it deserves some loving care? It works all day and night for you without stopping. What reward does it receive?

Your heart actually doesn't work as well if you don't give it something to do.

It's a *muscle,* after all. A man who is in top physical condition by exercising regularly will have a resting heart rate of about sixty beats per minute or less. A man who is not in good condition forces his heart to beat nearly thirty thousand times more every day of his life. If you are *out* of shape, your heart will beat proportionately faster than if you were *in* shape doing the same activity. And if your heart is not in shape, the rest of you is not in shape, either.

Dr. Kenneth Cooper has a good illustration describing your heart and how it works. He says the heart is like a "lawn with built-in watering jets or like one watered with a small garden hose. The hose might water the entire lawn eventually but, during a hot spell, it might take too long and some of the lawn might burn up. If part of your heart 'burned up' because it couldn't get enough sprinkling, it could mean a heart attack."

How to Know Your Pulse Rate

To know your resting pulse rate, take your resting pulse for one full minute once a week before getting out of bed in the morning. Write it down. As you enter the fitness program and make progress, you will notice your pulse rate lowering and leveling out. In the first few weeks it may rise a little, but don't worry. That is because your body is getting accustomed to hard work.

I will ask you to take your pulse in the middle of the aerobic section of your exercise. Here's how to do it: Place your four fingers at the side of your neck or on your wrist, and count the beat of your heart for only six seconds. Multiply that number by 10. If you come up with a count of 16 beats, for example, your heart rate is 16 times 10 or 160. This is an accurate indication of your peak-exercise pulse rate.

There is a handy formula for knowing if you are exercising too fast or too slow. The way to calculate this is what most exercise physiologists agree on. There are two types of exercise heart rates:

1. Minimum Exercise Heart Rate for those in average shape
2. Maximum Exercise Heart Rate for those who are becoming more fit

The formula is this: Your Minimum Exercise Heart Rate is 170 minus your age.

Your Maximum Exercise Heart Rate is 200 minus your age.

If your age is forty-four and your Minimum Exercise Heart Rate is 126, your Maximum Exercise Heart Rate would be

TABLE 1 OPTIMUM HEARTBEAT RATE DURING EXERCISE FOR WOMEN

AGE	MINIMUM WITH EXERCISE	MAXIMUM WITH EXERCISE	OPTIMUM OR 80% OF MAXIMUM HEART RATE
25	130	185	148
30	126	180	144
35	123	175	140
40	119	170	136
45	116	165	132
50	112	160	128
55	109	155	124
60	105	150	120
65	102	145	116

TABLE 2 OPTIMUM HEARTBEAT RATE DURING EXERCISE FOR MEN

AGE	MINIMUM WITH EXERCISE	MAXIMUM WITH EXERCISE	OPTIMUM OR 80% OF MAXIMUM HEART RATE
25	137	195	156
30	133	190	152
35	130	185	148
40	126	180	144
45	123	175	140
50	119	170	136
55	116	165	132
60	112	160	128
65	109	155	124

156. This means that if you are not in good shape, you shouldn't let your heart rate go any higher than 126 during exercise. Later on, as you become better conditioned, you can push for 156. Actually you could push for an even higher rate as you get more in shape, say up to 160. This is a formula that is very easy to remember and is an excellent guide, followed by virtually all fitness instructors. When I am exercising at my optimum, my heart rate usually pumps higher than my maximum because I am in fairly good condition.

In order for cardiovascular improvement to begin, you must reach your maximum heart rate while exercising. If you find your exercise sessions don't get you up to your maximum heart rate, increase the intensity with which you're doing your exercises, or the duration of them. Dr. Frank Katch, chairman of the exercise science department at the University of Massachusetts, has a system he calls FITT, which he designed as a model for getting our cardiovascular systems into shape.

- F means Frequency: Work out three to four days per week.
- I means Intensity: Work out at your top heart rate.
- T means Time: Exercise for a minimum of thirty minutes per session. (In our program we are starting with ten-minute periods if you're really out of shape, and increasing it gradually.)
- T means Type of Exercise: You will be doing exercises and aerobic activities that will work out your heart and lungs as well as utilize the muscle groups in your arms, legs, back, and abdomen.

Ben Jonson said that physical health is the blessing of the rich and the riches of the poor. Getting to know yourself and how your body functions is a great aid to physical health. Wonderfully created, your body will bless you if you bless it by caring for it. Herbert Spencer said that the preservation of health is a duty.

It's healthy to be in shape. Staying in shape requires your understanding your body. The next chapter will tell you what body type you have and more about how it works.

Dear Lord Jesus, Thank You for me and the body You've given me. Thank You for the opportunity to give You every fiber and tissue of my being so that being healthy will glorify You. Amen.

6

Your Body Type and Muscles

What Body Type Are You?

The psychology of relating body type to temperament is known as *constitutional psychology*. Its chief proponent has been William Sheldon, a physician as well as a psychologist. Sheldon's somatotypes and their personality traits are well known and placed in three general classifications. They are the *endomorph*, the *mesomorph*, and the *ectomorph*.

Sheldon proposes that when one of these dimensions predominates, we have an endomorph (fat and soft), a mesomorph (strong and athletic), or an ectomorph (tall and slender). By a rating procedure known as somatotyping, a person is scored on a seven-point scale to see which of these traits are most dominant in his or her physique. Almost no one fits a perfect description of one category alone.

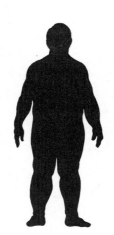

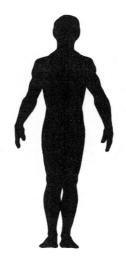

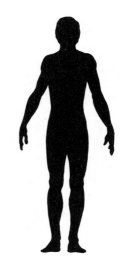

Endomorph	*Mesomorph*	*Ectomorph*
Inclined to be round and plump. The social, friendly type who likes to eat but who burns off calories slowly. Pounds add quickly and leave slowly, usually settling on the waist, hips, and thighs.	A large figure with big bones and a firm body. An athletic type who is energetic and tireless, with a good appetite. This person is usually aggressive and competitive, and his weight usually remains the same. Needs a strict diet and special spot exercises.	Slender by nature, with delicate body and long waist. Ectomorphs seldom gain more than a pound or two, no matter what they eat. They seem to burn up calories just sitting still. They are often socially inhibited, quick to react, and may have poor sleeping habits coupled with constant fatigue.

Are You Large or Small Boned?

You may weigh more than an ideal-weight chart says you should and still look tiny. Your bone structure tells you how much you should weigh. If you have large bones, you should weigh in at the heavy end of the recommended range for your height. To find out whether your bones are large or small, measure your wrist an inch above the bony part. Divide that into your height. If it goes more than twelve times, you probably have light bones; less than eleven times, your bones are on the heavy side.

Why Your Best Friends Should Be Your Muscles

God gave you muscles so you could have a blessed and happy life. Muscles are contractile tissues composed of fibrils, which shorten when chemically activated. Your muscles comprise 35 to 45 percent of your total body weight (remember that when you get on the scale).

You have three kinds of muscle:

Skeletal: under voluntary control (these are the ones *you* work)
Cardiac: found only in the heart
Smooth: as in the intestine (involuntary and controlled by the autonomic nervous system)

Now here's what happens. Your skeletal muscles are designed to *contract.* By contracting, they strengthen. Muscle tone is maintained when your fibrils are always being stimulated to contract.

Muscles come in pairs, like husband and wife, so that as one contracts the other slowly relaxes, to give a smooth, controlled movement. Muscles pull gently against each other and this is what we call *muscle tone*. They make beautiful music together.

Here's the good part: When your muscles contract, energy is required and heat produced. This makes a change (a metabolism) and it produces carbon dioxide, lactic acid, heat, and water. The blood flow into the muscles is increased to take away the metabolites, and your heart rate increases. The heat is dissipated through your skin by sweating. Get it?

What it all means is that when you exercise you make your muscles very happy and, after all, what are friends for?

You have more than 434 skeletal muscles responsible for every move you make. When you successfully stimulate fitness in the large-muscle groups, your minor-muscle groups are affected in the process. There are fifteen basic muscle groups, and when you give them a thorough workout, most of the 434 skeletal muscles will benefit. Here is a list of those fifteen marvelous muscles:

1. the lower back
2. the latissimus dorsi (the large, fanlike muscles that laterally cover most of your back)

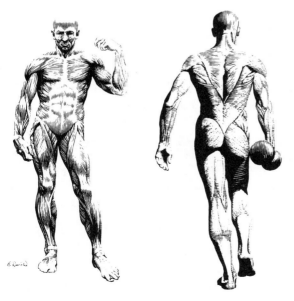

3. your deltoids (shoulder muscles)
4. pectorals (chest muscles)
5. trapezius (the muscles between the deltoids and the neck)
6. triceps (the muscles on the back of your upper arm)
7. biceps (the muscles on the front of your upper arm)
8. forearm (muscles on both sides of the forearm)
9. quadriceps (muscles on the front of the thigh)
10. biceps femoris (muscles at the back of the thigh, known as your hamstrings.
11. gluteus maximus (the muscle in your buttocks)
12. adductors (muscles on the inside of your thighs)
13. abductors (muscles on the outside of your thighs)
14. gastrocnemius (your calf muscles)
15. five abdominals (muscles at the front and sides of your trunk)

For most of the actions your body performs, your muscles are working together in order to do what you want done. Most muscles have more than one function. When you are just sitting or standing around, your muscles are constantly *contracting* (shortening) and *extending* (lengthening) to balance your body against the forces of gravity. These movements are automatic, and you don't have to consciously think about them to do them. You don't tell yourself, *Now I am going to lift my hand,* and *Now I am going to put it down again,* every time you lift and put your hand down. Nevertheless, those muscles of yours are constantly at work for you. They need your attention, however, because without it they do not function as they ought to.

I have listed for you the fifteen basic muscle groups, and now I want you to think about the five groups you will be concentrating on in this program. Starting from your head to your toes are:

Upper-Body Muscles

The muscles in your upper body include your *neck muscles,* which are responsible for moving your head from front to back and side to side and protecting your upper spinal cord from injury. Also included in your upper-body muscles are your *shoulder muscles.* This important group of muscles (your deltoids) covers your shoulders—top, sides, front, and back. Your neck muscles are important in sports such as soccer and wrestling, and your shoulder muscles are extremely important in sports such as tennis, golf, archery, and swimming. The deltoids are used in all of your daily activities which involve raising your arms.

Also in this muscle group are your *chest muscles.* You know about your pectoral muscles, which are located on the sides and center of your chest and underneath your breasts. When you lift, move, or push anything, you use your pectorals. Your breast tissue is supported by these muscles. Sports requiring pectoral strength are swimming, tennis, golf, and any sport requiring throwing.

Upper-back muscles are made up of two important muscle groups: the trapezius and latissimus dorsi. Most women have very weak lats, which is why we don't do well at chin-ups and rope climbing. You need both of these upper-back muscle groups in sports such as tennis, golf, swimming, rowing, fencing, and archery.

Arm Muscles

There are three muscles in your arms. The first is the back of your *upper arm.* This muscle is called the triceps and it makes up two-thirds of your upper arm. Like the lats, triceps are usually underdeveloped in most women, and that is why we tend to get flabby in the upper-arm area. You need your triceps to lift things

over your head or extend your arms in any direction.

In the front of the upper arm is your biceps. Its main purpose is to bend your elbow, and it is used in any lifting movement in which your arm is bent, and in any pulling movement. The biceps work together with your lats and deltoids. If you want to see your biceps in all its glory, stand in front of a mirror, make a fist with your arm bent, and flex. Don't you feel strong?

Forearm muscles. The muscles of your forearm are responsible for moving your wrist and for gripping. Grip is important. Racket sports, golf, handball, fishing, and baseball need the strength of your forearm muscles. (They also come in handy for hailing a cab, chopping celery, and playing the harp!)

Abdominal Muscles

Your abdominal muscles are located in the center and along the sides of your abdomen. These very important muscles aid in your posture, in stabilizing your trunk during activity, and holding your internal organs in place. It is vital that these muscles be in shape. Countless disorders are due to lack of use of these muscles. Your abdominal muscles are used in all activities and all sports. Your new program will shape up your abdominal muscles beautifully.

Hip and Lower-Back Muscles

Running is a good way to strengthen your lower-back muscles, which is one of the most ignored muscle groups of the body. Like the abdominal muscles, the lower-back muscles are necessary in every one of your daily activities. They are extremely important in maintaining posture.

Leg Muscles

The four muscle groups here begin with the *buttocks.* This is an area of the body where women carry excess body fat. Underneath the fat is the largest and strongest muscle group of your entire body. The purpose of the buttocks muscle is to move your thighs. Conditioned buttocks muscles are essential for walking, running, and are used in sports such as skiing, skating, swimming, biking, football, and soccer.

The muscle at the *front of the thigh* is the quadriceps, and its main function is to straighten your knees. People with knee problems often have weak quadriceps.

The muscle group located on the *back of your thigh* is called the hamstring. The hamstring's main function is to bend your knee. This muscle group is important in all physical exercises. Tight hamstrings are sometimes a major cause of lower-back pain. This is especially common in people who don't exercise.

Calf muscles are located on the back of your lower legs. Their main purpose is to lift your heels off the floor. Without them, you wouldn't be able to walk. Women suffer from shortened, inflexible calf muscles, which sometimes cause ankle pain because of years of wearing high-heeled shoes. Your calves are vitally important in any daily activity which requires mobility.

In order to develop your muscles, you want to be sure to work *all* of them. Most of us tend to be weaker in certain muscles than in others, and our daily activities develop strength and endurance in different areas of our bodies. If you run every day, you will have strength in your legs and cardiovascular strength, but chances are you will be weak when it comes to lifting. Your upper body will not be as strong proportionately as your lower body.

Golf is a good exercise for the caddy. As far as its being sufficient as your sole source of physical exercise, it is sadly lacking. You walk slowly, and the stroke used in golf is always from one side, leaving the other side of the body unexercised. There is very little stretching the muscles of the lower body.

One young mother of four told me she got plenty of exercise during the day by running up and down stairs, doing the laundry, cooking, and taking care of her demanding family. Actually she was not getting enough exercise, because her muscles were not being developed to their maximum. You may think you get enough exercise if your daily work is physical, but you are not. Say, for instance, you work as a waiter. Just because you are on your feet all day and moving quickly does not guarantee that you will have strength in the five muscle groups we have named. You need a balanced exercise program to be strong in all areas of your body.

After examining the parts of your body, you can certainly gain a greater insight into the joy of the Word: "In every thing give thanks: for this is the will of God in Christ Jesus concerning you" (1 Thessalonians 5:18).

Let's you and I praise the Lord together and rejoice that we can glorify God by being strong and healthy for Him.

For ye are bought with a price: therefore glorify God in your body, and in your spirit, which are God's.

1 Corinthians 6:20

7

What Are You Eating?

The Best Diet for You

How can I make you understand that those candy bars you have hidden under the seat of the car simply are *not* good for you? I have a friend Myrna, who told me at one time, "I'd eat nails if they were chocolate covered." She told me how she hid chocolate behind her Tupperware in the cupboard until her kids found it. "You're supposed to be on a diet!" they shrieked at her.

"I *am* on a diet," she argued back.

"But what's this?" they accused, pointing to telltale empty candy wrappers in the half-gallon juice container behind the mixing bowls and plastic sandwich boxes.

"Those? How should I know? Maybe the last people who lived in this house left them there."

Myrna was so guilt ridden, she went out and had a hot-fudge sundae to calm her nerves.

She tried everything to lose weight. She went on the grapefruit-and-egg diet, the fruit diet, the water diet, the fish diet, the Stillman diet, the Scarsdale diet, the Atkins diet, the Beverly Hills diet. She took Metrecal, liquid protein, Slenderall, diet pills, diet candies and wafers, diuretics, not to mention enemas. She fasted, bought creams, belts, girdles guaranteed to "whittle away fat while sleeping," and *still* she carried around twenty-five pounds of extra weight. She joined a health spa but was too self-conscious to be seen so fat in front of all those other people.

One day she read my book *Free to be Thin*, which tells of the Overeaters Victorious weight loss method. She lost every pound of excess weight. How? She learned to listen to the Lord tell her how to eat. She realized that the Lord really cared about her and about her weight problem. She found out, also, that the Lord is really sensible when it comes to food. In John 6:1–13, the Lord Jesus was preaching to two thousand people and at lunchtime there was nothing for them to eat, so He miraculously and marvelously multiplied one little boy's lunch of bread and fish to feed all those people, with enough left over to fill twelve baskets. Can you just imagine Him feeding all those people that day on a box of Ayds and black coffee?

You're going to have fun being fit and in shape, so I want you to look at what you're putting into your body with real earnest concern.

The Most Important Diet Tip in This Book

Think Blood Sugar Level. It's when your blood sugar level is low that you want to eat. That's when you crave the chocolate-covered nails. Anything sweet and gooey gives you a quick-energy blood sugar high with a sudden shot of glucose in the blood. Then *zingo,* the pancreas starts overproducing insulin and the old blood sugar takes a plunge. Insulin is quick acting, and then the glucose level drops sharply. There you are, back where you started. Low blood sugar creates intense hunger (a craving for more sweets) so you're back in the cupboard, opening lids on your Tupperware like a wild maniac, looking for that cache of chocolate.

Low blood sugar also creates irritability, moodiness, and depression. You pacify these emotions temporarily with food. Sweets, if you can get your pudgy little hands on some, will do the trick, but there you are again, in the same predicament you started with. Your blood sugar rises after you eat the sugary food, then it falls, *plop.* The cycle goes on. You're getting fatter by the day.

Complex carbohydrates release glucose gradually, so they don't do you in.

Learn to eat foods that will stabilize your blood sugar level. That way you will not gorge or eat the wrong foods. If you can cold-turkey the sugar, white flour, and processed foods, you'll be blessing yourself beyond your dreams.

The secret of getting thin and staying there is to keep your blood sugar stable. I know I am repeating myself, but it's one of my best tips. Get to know your body. When do you like to eat the most? (Yes, I know, "all the time," silly, but there are times of the day when you are inclined to eat *more.*)

When you find yourself craving something sweet, eat an orange or an apple to get your blood sugar up. Stay away from the no-nos, and I don't have to tell you what they are—except for one little no-no you may not be so aware of. It's coffee. Coffee triggers a yo-yo effect with your blood sugar. It has somewhat the same effect on your body as refined carbohydrates, because it accelerates the blood sugar to a false energy high. Then it drops it to an all-time low, leaving you feeling irritable, moody, depressed, and wanting something to eat. Many nutritionists claim coffee is a definite *deterrent* to weight control.

One mistake we often make when trying to lose weight is that we cut out fat from the diet altogether. You need a little fat, but you need the right kind. The best sources of fat are *polyunsaturated* ones which lower cholesterol. You get them in fish and safflower, corn, and cottonseed oils. Nutritionist Dr. N. Walker claims raw avocado or alligator pear and olive oil are the best-quality fat for the body. He claims nothing cooked in fat is good for you. Try "air popping" your popcorn the next time, and remember, no french-fried potato is a friend of yours.

I should mention cigarette smoking and alcohol so you can be glad you don't use either. They not only age you and bloat you but they also give you wrinkles, cellulite, and broken blood vessels, and they destroy your body and kill your brain cells. God delivers us from destruction (Psalms 103:4), and we can thank God we're delivered from the ravages of the use of cigarettes, drugs, and alcohol on our precious bodies. For most of us, drinking is not a problem. It's those cakes and cookies that have a way of finding their way into our mouths.

Let's say you conquered the "sin of the sweet tooth." Let's say you haven't had anything sugary in over a month, and not only that, it has been ages since a thick, fattening pastrami sandwich crossed your lips. (Just because it's protein doesn't mean it's right.) But you weigh the same as you did last summer.

"I starve myself and *still* can't lose weight!" you sigh wistfully, and somewhat accusingly, at me. *"Why don't I lose weight?"*

After telling me how you've read *Free to Be Thin* seventeen times, and how you haven't touched anything but cottage cheese and lettuce all week, I'm beginning to be suspicious.

"How much cottage cheese?"

"What's that got to do with anything?"

"Aha!" I respond knowingly. "The case is solved. You're eating *too much* cottage cheese and whatever else you're putting in your mouth."

You may be eating only sprouted mung beans and watermelon, but I guarantee you, it's no way to lose weight and keep it off. You can't eat an entire watermelon at one sitting and lose weight! Remember your blood sugar level. What happens in another couple of hours? Your stomach is stretched, your tissues drenched, and you're starved.

Tracy R., one of the ladies in a Free to Be Thin group at the Christian Center for Counseling and Fitness, complained how she only ate yogurt, chicken, salads, fresh fruit, and wheat germ all week and *still* didn't lose a pound. It turned out she ate an entire chicken at a clip, a half cup of wheat germ mixed in her eight ounces of yogurt a few times a day, and her salads had at least a third of a cup of dressing on each one. For fruit she ate three or four bananas, apples, and as many as six oranges at a time. By the end of the day she was putting away over twenty-five hundred calories. You don't lose weight on twenty-five hundred calories unless you happen to be something equivalent to a small rhinoceros.

It's important that you weigh and measure what you eat. Please get to know what a half cup of something looks like. Weigh your meat and chicken. Almost every diet you read says things like, "three ounces of chicken," "eight ounces of juice," "a half cup of vegetable," and other such instructions. I have a postage scale on my kitchen counter, and I advise you to put one on yours, too. You would be amazed how small a half cup of zabaglione really is.

Weight Loss Bell Ringers

Rather than suggest diets or give you food plans, let me give you some tips (although the blood sugar one is the best one yet) that will really help you drop extra pounds.

1. Be prepared for the "Wild Munchies." When you're suddenly seized with an uncontrollable urge to munch (and munch and munch), have fresh vegetables all sliced and waiting in a nice little plastic bag in the refrigerator.

2. Here's a chance to use that Tupperware as something other than a place to hide your midnight fudge in. Cut up crisp salad yummies like romaine lettuce, raw sliced turnips, zucchini or summer squash, jicama, green peppers, carrots, and mushrooms. Keep these in the

front of the shelf in your refrigerator. When it's meal time, you have a "fast food" just waiting for you. All you have to do is open your salad delight and top it with something fabulous like a dollop of yogurt or cottage cheese. Then, on top of that, sprinkle some dry roasted soybeans, sesame or sunflower seeds, raisins, bran, and wheat germ. Heaven!

3. Think raw. Medical researchers say our health is in trouble when we don't eat enough whole, uncooked foods. Temperatures over 130° F. kill enzymes which are naturally contained in food to help with the digestion and absorption of the nutrients. Vitamins are lost in cooking. As much as 60 percent of vitamin C in vegetables disappears during cooking. Vegetables lose 25 to 40 percent of their B vitamins in cooking. Essential minerals are also lost in the cooking water. Raw is the best way to serve fruits and vegetables. Stir frying and steaming are second best because they are quick-cooking methods.

4. Don't overcook meat. Meat loses 35 percent of its vitamin B_1, 20 percent of its B_2, and 25 percent of its niacin in cooking.

5. The American Medical Association says that food quackery is the most profitable form of charlatanry in the United States. It claims that $500 million a year is spent by the public on reducing pills, cure-all food supplements, and other weight loss schemes. Keep your money and understand that the only way to lose weight is to stop eating more than you need and to exercise.

6. Realize, as you face that bakery window, that what you *really* want is not that ugly pastry. You know in your heart it is not what will *really* comfort you if you're feeling depressed or unloved. Having a fattening, sugary blob of pastry rolling around in your stomach is not really what will fill the emptiness you're feeling. Go next door to the delicatessen and buy an orange. Then go home, call a Christian friend, and get blessed!

7. Stop using going out to restaurants as an opportunity to overeat. There's hardly a restaurant around where you can't find broiled fish *sans* butter, or an omelet. How about plain roast beef or baked chicken (don't eat the skin)? And the blessed salad bar! You can always make yourself a marvelous salad and people won't even realize you're watching your weight.

8. Restaurants to avoid while losing weight:
   German. No matter what anybody says, those dumplings will only "dumple" your midriff. Of course, if sauerkraut is your thing, you're okay here. Eat as much as you like and you won't gain weight.
   French. Can you resist the sauces?
   Mexican. Unless you only eat the shredded lettuce of your taco.

9. I should include Italian in the above list of restaurants to avoid, but who can live without Italian food? Take my house and my car, but don't take away Italian food! How cruel can you be? I've cunningly devised a way to eat Italian food and still eat slim (no, not bulimia). I never eat the pasta, only the sauce, and half or a quarter of it at that. I don't touch the bread, and eat all meats broiled only with garlic and spices. I order vegetables without butter. *Mamma mia,* I'm clever.
   Yes: Roast peppers
   Broiled shrimp (scampi style, but *senza* butter)
   Clams marinara
   Zuppa de pesce (fish soup)
   Veal pailland
   Chicken cacciatore

10. Restaurants to frequent often:
    Chinese and Japanese. Lots of low-calorie veggie, fish, and meat dishes. Delicious stir-fry food without much oil. Stay away from the sauces and the monosodium glutamate. Eating with chopsticks is a definite plus because no matter how ravenous you are, the chopsticks will only pick up so much food at a time.

Natural Food Restaurants. Go wild on the salads and gourmet diet dishes. But remember to count calories. Some of the dishes are not for the slim-minded, although they may be incredibly nutritious.

11. If you're going to a place of temptation (like a good Italian restaurant), plan for it. Carefully think ahead and plan your calorie expenditure. Keep in mind that if you starve all day, your blood sugar level will be way down by dinner time and you could ruin your effort by taking a nose dive into the parmigiana. Keep your blood sugar steady during the day with fresh fruit and fresh fruit juices, a fresh salad for lunch, a glass of juice before dinner, and you'll be fine.

12. A word about fast-food hamburger and chicken places, hot dog stands, rib joints, and fast-food chain restaurants. Don't even inhale in these places. Look the other way when you pass by. The very lettuce in these places is fattening because it's drowned in mayo and catsup. You also could die of malnutrition here. And a deluxe hamburger has 950 calories. Who can afford it?

Why Results Take Time

So you're eating small portions, counting every calorie, and you haven't lost an ounce all week. There are many reasons for not losing weight, and they bear repeating. First, muscle weighs more than fat, and water in the tissues weighs something, too. You will retain more water at certain times of the month, such as just before your menstrual period begins. If you are eating less and eating better as we described here, you're going to lose weight. It may take longer than you want it to, but you *will* lose weight.

I joined a contest once to see who could lose the most percentage of weight in one month. How I starved! I thought for sure I would win that contest. On the day we weighed in, I re-

ceived the disappointing news that someone else had won the contest who had actually not even lost as much weight as I had. I was crushed in my defeat. I ran—not walked, *ran*—to my favorite Italian restaurant and—oh, I can't talk about it. But that's not all. Later, I rolled myself home, where I discovered a container of forbidden ice cream in the freezer. (I rue the day man discovered praline pecan, let me tell you.) The "Wild Munchies" had me in their evil grip, and—I shouldn't really discuss it in mixed company—suffice it to say, the freezer never saw that ice cream again, and in two days I gained six pounds. It took me *six weeks* to get it off!

Nobody has to lecture me on the wisdom of taking time to lose weight. It may be frustrating to stay at the same weight for several days, even when you're staying on your strict eating program, but it will be a glorious, lasting effect. The weight will stay off because your mind is set on losing weight, staying in shape, and glorifying God with your body.

If you feel tempted to overeat or to ruin your body by binging, just imagine me standing there beside you, whispering in your ear how your body will need four thousand extra feet of blood vessels to supply nourishment to one pound of fat. (I'd say more, but I'll leave that to the Lord.)

God has made something beautiful in your life, and still you're complaining, "If I just smell food or look at a pastry, I gain weight." Dr. Judith Rodin, a psychologist at Yale University, demonstrated how sight or smell of good food can actually affect metabolism. When Dr. Rodin analyzed blood samples of hungry volunteers who watched a steak being grilled with the promise that they would eat it, she discovered that overweight people reacted to the mere sight and smell of the food by producing greatly increased amounts of insulin. Insulin both stimulates the appetite and causes more of what we eat to be stored as fat. That may not be good news, but it's a word of caution to you. Try not to be around tempting foods when you're hungry. Remember your blood sugar level. Eat an orange, some raisins, or some natural fruit carboydrates before going to the supermarket.

If you're not losing weight, check your salt intake. Doctors tell us overuse of salt (sodium chloride) is not good for us. One-fourth teaspoon of extra salt can retain a half pound of water in our bodies. Using too much salt can harden the arteries and lead to hypertension, so the next time you reach for those salted peanuts, slap your hand and have a gorgeous carrot stick or juicy apple.

I know I don't have to discuss fad diets with a smart person like you, but I will anyhow. I hope you will avoid fad diets forever and ever. Amen. Fad diets really don't do you any good in the long run. Here's one I devised and believe me, a diet like this one really won't do what you think it will:

Emergency diet when your high school best friend calls from Walla Walla after ten years and says she'll be in town in twenty-four hours:
Breakfast: Juice of one lemon in warm water
Lunch: A pickle
Dinner: Four sections of a grapefruit

Don't tell me you've never starved yourself for some special event. We had a high school reunion last summer and at the end of the evening, one of the girls said, "Thank goodness it's over. Now I can *eat* again!"

You were set free from crash diets, fad diets, and destructive eating habits when the Lord Jesus died on the cross for your sins.

For	He gave you
your destructive choices	good works
impatience	long-suffering
self-hate	love and mercy
nervousness	peace and contentment
overeating problems	forgiveness and self-understanding
lack of self-control	power over the flesh
guilt	freedom and trust
shame	dignity

The purpose of Jesus' going to the cross was to set you free from the power of the devil. Jesus paid the price necessary for you to be free from destruction, negativity, and death. He paid the price for every sin in your life. He gave you His Spirit to overcome demonic forces as well as your negative choices and behaviors. Take your freedom.

Then he turned my sorrow into joy! He took away my clothes of mourning and gave me gay and festive garments to rejoice in so that I might sing glad praises to the Lord instead of lying in silence in the grave. O Lord my God, I will keep on thanking you forever!

Psalms 30:11,12 TLB

Bless yourself when you get on your scale. Say these words out loud: "I bless my spirit, soul, and body today in the name of Jesus. I refuse to be disconsolate. I am willing to allow God to bless me. I see a beautiful tomorrow."

8

The Program

Getting in Shape

Not long ago I brought a typewriter to the typewriter repair shop to be fixed. All of the keys stuck and the machine wouldn't type. The keyboard was locked tight, unable to function the way it was supposed to. The owner of the shop asked me, "When was the last time you used this machine?" I thought for a moment and then answered, "This machine probably hasn't been used in over a year."

"That's why it's in the shape it's in."

Our bodies are like that typewriter. If we don't use our bodies for a long time, they begin to lose their ability to do what they're designed to do. It used to be that physical inactivity was not listed as one of man's chief problems. Now, however, our lives have more stress and less physical activity than ever before. You must be aware from this very moment on that physical exercise is to be an

important part of your life if your body machinery is going to run smoothly.

The best kind of physical activity for your body is aerobic exercise. This demands oxygen in order for your lungs to process more air with less effort, thereby making your heart stronger and able to pump more blood with fewer strokes, so that the blood supply to your muscle improves and your total blood volume increases.

Why Aerobics?

Aerobic exercises are a variety of exercises such as running, jumping, and swimming to stimulate the heart and lung activity for a long period of time to produce significant changes in your body. With aerobics, your lungs, heart, and vascular system all benefit, as well as your muscles and bones.

Aerobic literally means "with oxygen." Aerobic exercise causes your cardiorespiratory system—your heart, lungs, and blood vessels—to operate more efficiently. They are better able to take oxygen from the air, process it, and deliver it to your muscles and organs. When you're in shape, your cardiorespiratory system has less work to do in order to keep your body running well.

Your heart is going to love you for your new getting-in-shape program. You're going to breathe easier because the muscles in your chest will grow stronger, and you will be able to breathe air in and out of your lungs with less effort.

You will reduce your risk of heart disease, heart attack, and stroke. You don't have to be a marathon runner to achieve these excellent results. *Any* increase in your level of physical activity will make you more fit. It doesn't matter what shape you're in now, how old you are, or how long it's been since you were physically active. Anyone can be fit, have a healthier heart, and bless his body. Please be sure to check with your physician before you engage in any physical fitness program. Be sure you have his okay.

To get the most from your aerobics program, it must include the following important components:

Frequency of Exercise

A minimum of three days per week, preferably on alternate days. Maximum: six days a week. Your body needs one day to rest.

Duration of Exercise

Twenty to thirty minutes spent in aerobic conditioning with a goal of continuous, steady activity. This can be done slowly, with five-minute durations, and building up the time each exercise period.

Intensity of Exercise

You will want to reach 60 to 80 percent of your projected maximum heart rate. Remember, your maximal heart rate is approximately 200 minus your age.

Are You Breathing?

That's a silly question, isn't it? Of course you're breathing, or you wouldn't be reading this book. The important matter here is, are you breathing correctly? In your active daily breathing, you draw air into your lungs by the action of your diaphragm, which is a muscle that looks something like a piece of rubber sheeting that stretches across your chest and separates your chest cavity from your abdomen.

When you inhale fresh oxygen, it must make contact with the blood in the lungs. When you inhale, you bring fresh oxygen into contact with your old, used blood, and this happens through the walls of your hairlike blood vessels. These vessels are thick enough to contain blood and also thin enough to allow the oxygen to penetrate them. When the oxygen contacts the blood, the blood takes up the good, fresh oxygen for your body, and at the same time gets rid of the carbon dioxide gas which has been gathered from all the parts of your body in toxins and waste matter. Your blood is then purified and oxygenated and ready to bless your body.

I'm giving you this fascinating study in physiology just so you can see how important it is to breathe correctly. The way you breathe makes a big difference. Shallow breathing brings only a portion of your lung cells into play, and your body has been underoxygenated.

Give yourself this little test: Stand up and take a deep breath. Notice whether your shoulders are raised and your breath is up at the base of your throat. If this is so, you are engaging in shallow breathing.

Another way of breathing shallowly is to swell out your chest as you inhale. You are using only about half of your lungs' capacity when you take a deep breath this way.

The correct way to breathe is to use your diaphragm, the muscle covering the abdomen in an arc and protruding into your chest cavity. Your diaphragm will expand when your lower lungs are filled. In deep breathing, your stomach will appear to swell down and out. Opera singers are masters at deep breathing. (My Uncle Fred was an opera singer. You ought to see him breathe.)

Try another breath now, this time with your hands on your stomach. Take a deep breath and feel your stomach expand. If you practice this often, you will be filling your lungs and raising the oxygen level of your blood to an energetic high point. You will also be aiding in the expulsion of toxins and wastes.

Before deep breathing you will want to exhale. That way you are getting rid of impurities first.

Breathing properly is essential to your health because your cells need oxygen. Oxygen combined with glucose (or the body's fuel) in your bloodstream forms energy. Anything you do that interferes with your body's processes of oxygenation and the removal of carbon dioxide will cause your cells to slowly become exhausted. The reason overweight people often breathe heavily is that their lungs are not able to increase in size to match the rest of them. They must struggle to get the necessary oxygen to their extra fat cells.

Extra fat around your abdomen will restrict your breathing. Air sacs in your lungs can become infiltrated with fat and cut down on the volume of air your lungs can handle.

Exercise is vital to your respiration.

The oxygen capacity of your lungs increases with exercise, and stored fat is used up.

You may have a tendency to hold your breath while exercising. Don't do it. You need to get the oxygen into your bloodstream. You also need to breathe out to eliminate the waste products and toxic gases. *As a general rule, breathe out when you're making the most effort, and breathe in when you ease up.* In each of the exercises I'm going to give you I will indicate the proper breathing. It's important to follow these directions.

It is always best to exercise on an empty stomach. After you eat, your heart pumps extra blood to your stomach to help in the digestive process, and if you exercise on a full stomach, the blood doesn't know which way to go. It will go to your muscles and deprive your stomach of oxygen. That's why you become nauseous or cramped.

You can drink water during your exercise. It won't hurt you. When you're finished exercising, drink orange juice or natural fruit juice to replenish your supply of potassium and trace minerals.

Physiologists say it only takes three to four weeks to become unconditioned, even if you start out fit. If you go off your exercise routine for a week or longer, begin again slowly and at a lower level of intensity. Your muscles will have lost some of their ability to use oxygen efficiently, so you want to be good to them and help them recover.

Commitment Is Everything

You are making a firm commitment when you begin this life-changing program. Occasional jogging is not enough to bless your body. One aerobics class a week is not enough to help you in all the ways we have discussed. Weekend tennis is not enough in itself, and neither is ten minutes a day of calisthenics.

This is not a short-term program you are embarking upon, but a lifetime one. You are going to work your heart and lungs for the rest of your life. Think of this time of your day as natural and *absolutely necessary.* Your exercise program will be done six days a week. Plan on it. Once again, six days a week.

If you have not exercised strenuously for several years, or if you are more than twenty-five pounds overweight, or if you have a serious medical history and are over forty years old, please make an appointment with your doctor for a thorough examination before starting to exercise. Your examination should include an electrocardiogram (EKG) taken at rest.

If exercising six days a week sounds like too much for you, don't force yourself. Remember that it's *fun* to be fit and it's fun to get that way. Start with exercising three times a week, and gradually work up to six. Jacki Sorensen, the director and originator of Aerobic Dancing, Inc., says that you must do your aerobic dancing at least three times a week if you want to be physically fit. Aerobic dancing or any aerobic-type activity will do.

If you're out of shape, don't worry about huffing and puffing at your workouts. As long as you aren't dizzy, nauseous, fainting, or blacking out, you're all right. It's important to take your pulse at the specific times you are instructed to so you know what's going on with your body. A rule of thumb is to avoid pushing yourself too hard, but on the other hand push yourself enough to challenge your body. As I said before, you want to make sweating your goal. You will push yourself a little beyond what you think you can do. You'll be amazed at the energy and strength you have trapped in that wonderful body of yours.

When you begin the program, you will be reading the instructions and looking at the pictures as you exercise. Read the instructions carefully so that you do the exercises correctly. After several sessions you will have memorized the exercises and won't need to have the book in front of you. Each exercise is designed to flow from one to the other without pausing in between. Become familiar with these exercises, even though it takes a little more time at the beginning.

You can do these exercises alone or with a friend. They are the same ones we are doing in our classes. The wonderful benefit of a program such as this book offers is that all you need is the book. You do not need to invest in expensive exercise equipment, spas, or fancy exercise clothing. All you need is you, a little space, and determination.

At first you may be stiff after exercising, and you can minimize this by getting into a hot bath after your workout, before your muscles have cooled down. Don't stop exercising when you are stiff, because continuing to exercise will dissipate the stiffness. It only lasts a week or so anyhow. You may also experience muscle swelling in the beginning, but don't worry about it. It's because you're working your muscles so hard and they are so surprised by it, they react by swelling somewhat. Any kind of pain you feel should be listened to and identified. The healthy pain which comes from any vigorous physical exertion is a good pain. Know your body.

One of my students came to me after class one day complaining of a sore foot. She was afraid she had torn something. After looking at it, we saw the problem was she had laced her sneakers too tightly! After becoming accustomed to exercising, you will recognize the different kinds of pains in your body, and which ones tell you there's something wrong. I believe the Lord Jesus will bless you and bless your body. He has said He will give you the desires of your heart, and if it is your desire to be fit and faithful to being fit, He will grant you your desire. Be sure you do not allow yourself to expect anything less than God's best, because that's what He gives you.

Remember to go to the bathroom *before* you start exercising. You don't want to have to leave in the middle of it and ruin your momentum.

Take the phone off the hook when you start to exercise.

Get yourself a place in the house where you will exercise every day. It should be somewhere without a draft, with a ceiling high enough to allow you to jump up and clap your hands over your head. You also want enough space to swing your arms wide without hitting anything. The space between your coffee table and living-room sofa just won't do.

You need an exercise pad or a heavy carpet under you when you exercise. You may also want to put a towel on top of the carpet. Do not do the aerobic part of your program barefoot. Always wear your sneakers. The sneakers should be of the finest quality. Don't buy those $1.98 rubber specials you find on bargain tables at discount stores. Your body needs the support and cushioning of an excellent pair of shoes designed for aerobic exercise. Even if your feet and legs are in perfect shape, don't do your aerobic exercises barefoot. The rest of the program you may do without shoes, but not jumping. Never run barefoot unless you're on the beach and not going to run for more than a mile or so. You may step on something and cut your feet, or strain your feet seriously.

Get yourself a logbook to record your daily workout. This will include your frequency, duration, and intensity, as well as your resting pulse rate. I also record my weight at the beginning of each week.

The Importance of Keeping a Log

I keep my log as a chart taped on the inside of my kitchen cupboard. At the end of each of my fitness sessions, I go to my chart and fill it in. Some people keep their fitness chart alongside their calorie-counting chart so they can maintain control over both of these things at the same time. This log is crucial because you will be watching your own improvement before your very eyes. Also, you will receive a wonderful feeling at the end of the week when you see your chart filled, representing your faithful adherence to your program. I take my chart with me when I go out of town and tape it on the inside of my suitcase so I can continue to keep it up-to-date. No matter what, do not forget to record on your fitness chart every single day, even if it's to enter a zero for that day. Your log might look something like the one on page 64.

You will be giving yourself points for each activity on the program. A check after Workout, for example, means you accomplished full workout on the program, including the warm-up and cool-down, as well as the stretches and calisthenics. Each check is equal to two points. When you check Aerobic Exercise, give yourself two points for each five minutes of exercise. If you run for ten minutes, for example, you will receive two checks, or four points. Riding your stationary bicycle for thirty minutes would be equivalent to twelve points.

By using this system, you can more efficiently gauge your progress. It is not meant to be a scientific study. It is simply a means of observing your progress. As you can see by the scoring chart

COMPUTING YOUR DAILY POINTS
WEEK OF ____

BEGINNING WEIGHT ____   ENDING WEIGHT ____   RESTING HEART RATE ____

Activity	MONDAY Duration: Intensity:	Points	TUESDAY Duration: Intensity:	Points	WEDNESDAY Duration: Intensity:	Points	THURSDAY Duration: Intensity:	Points	FRIDAY Duration: Intensity:	Points	SATURDAY Duration: Intensity:	Points	SUNDAY Duration: Intensity:	Points
Workout														
Aerobic Exercise														
Running														
Tennis														
Racquetball														
Ice/Roller Skating														
Bicycling														
Jumping Rope														
Rebound Jumping														

TOTAL POINTS: ____

TOTAL WEEKLY POINTS: ____
TOTAL RUNNING HOURS: ____
TOTAL WORKOUT HOURS: ____
TOTAL AEROBIC HOURS: ____

SCORING YOURSELF

ACTIVITY COMPLETE	POINTS	DURATION
Workout	2	for each 5 minutes (warm-up, stretch, calisthenics, cool-down)
Aerobic Exercise	2	for each 5 minutes vigorous exercise
Running	2	for each 5 minutes running at vigorous pace
Tennis (singles)	2	for each 10 minutes
(doubles)	2	for each 15 minutes
Racquetball	2	for each 10 minutes continual activity
Ice/Roller Skating	2	for each 15 minutes continual movement at vigorous pace
Bicycling (stationery)	2	for each 5 minutes nonstop
(out-of-doors)	2	for each 15 minutes nonstop
Jumping Rope	2	for each 5 minutes
Rebound Jumping	2	for each 10 minutes

above, you can earn as many as fifty or sixty points a week right in the beginning. Each week you will be adding more and more points. As your condition improves, it's quite possible to work up to two hundred, even three hundred points or more a week.

The following is a chart to show you some aerobic activities and their benefits:

AEROBIC ACTIVITIES AND THEIR BENEFITS

ACTIVITIES	BENEFITS
Running:	Cardiovascular fitness, lowers body fat percentage faster than all other aerobic activities. If you run one mile in less than ten minutes, you are running. More than ten minutes and you are jogging.
Swimming:	Best cardiovascular conditioning exercise there is. No twisted ankles or blisters. Exercises all muscle groups and instead of muscle bulk, builds long, lean muscles. A vigorous swim will burn as many as five hundred calories in half an hour.
Skipping Rope:	Develops and strengthens calves, deltoids, and forearms. Tones quadriceps and hamstrings, abdominals, pectorals, lats, and biceps. Good overall aerobic workout.
Rebound Jumping:	Improves the heart and lungs and strengthens legs. Helps eliminate excess fat.
Skiing (downhill):	Waist, abdomen, and thighs strengthened. Excellent cardiovascular workout.
(cross-country):	Arm, shoulder, waist, abdomen, buttocks, calf, and ankle muscles strengthened. Cardiovascular workout better than most aerobic activities.
Racquetball and Handball:	Cardiovascular fitness. Improves reaction time, builds strength and stamina. Tones muscles, eliminates excess fat. You burn up to eight hundred calories an hour.
Bicycling:	Strengthens and tones thighs, calves, forearms, and gluteal muscles. Heart and lungs work more efficiently; circulation is improved. Helps control weight.
Tennis:	Develops muscles in one arm, strengthens quadriceps and buttocks. Develops agility and endurance; increases heart and lung strength.

All of these activities will bless your body. They're fun to do and you'll find yourself looking forward to them. My friend Marilyn learned the fun of aerobic activity when she learned to play tennis. Then she was in a devastating car accident and doctors told her chances of her ever playing tennis again were slim. She exercised and worked hard building her strength. In five months she was playing tennis. Just last week she won a championship in tennis through her tennis-club competition. She told me, "Marie, I believe God used tennis in my life to bring a healing to my body as well as my mind. After my accident I was miserable. All those broken bones. My right hand was paralyzed. I lay in bed all day feeling sorry for myself."

Marilyn radiated enthusiasm as she continued, "I decided to stop feeling sorry for myself. Instead I prayed for strength. I wanted to learn how to play tennis and I prayed God would give me the inner strength to work toward that goal. He answered that prayer. I can honestly say now I've never felt better in my life. Winning the tennis championship was like a gift from the Lord. It was His saying to me, *We made it!*"

Marilyn made it. You will, too. And you'll have fun as you do it.

Dear Jesus, Thank You for the strength to be more than I have ability to be. Thank You for Your power and Your love that breathes life and vigor into my whole being. Thank You for repairing me and lifting me out of the doldrums of self-centeredness. Thank You for fitness and thank You for loving me. Amen.

9

Benefits of Fitness

A Fitness Test

The Royal Canadian Air Force Exercise Plans for Physical Fitness includes the following four reasons you should be fit:

1. The physically fit person is able to withstand fatigue for longer periods than the unfit.
2. The physically fit person is better equipped to tolerate physical stress.
3. The physically fit person has a stronger and more efficient heart.
4. There is a relationship between good mental alertness, absence of nervous tension, and physical fitness.

With these in mind, answer these questions with as much honesty as you can. Remember, lying is frowned upon in heaven.

1. When you think of Thanksgiving Day, your first thought is of food.
_____True _____False
2. When you finish the food on your plate, you pick food off someone else's plate next to you.
_____True _____False
3. When you carry your suitcases in an airport, you nearly succumb to either a heart attack or physical collapse.
_____True _____False
4. You have absolutely no idea what might be behind your refrigerator because you never moved it to see.
_____True _____False
5. You always look for a parking place closest to the door of the supermarket so you don't have to walk far.
_____True _____False
6. You're convinced that most movie stars are beautiful, not because they exercise but because they were either born that way or they had extensive plastic surgery.
_____True _____False
7. You'd rather go to a new restaurant and eat than learn a new sport such as tennis or racquetball.
_____True _____False

8. You firmly believe that such activities as ice skating and ballet are only for an elite few.

    _____True _____False

9. When you go to sleep at night you sleep peacefully and wake up rested.

    _____True _____False

10. You rarely suffer any muscular aches and pains such as lower-back pain or neck-and-shoulder pain.

    _____True _____False

11. Your children find it hard to keep up with you because of your amazing physical endurance and agility.

    _____True _____False

12. You are perfectly satisfied with the way you look and feel at this moment.

    _____True _____False

13. You are usually hungriest at night and do most of your eating in the evening hours.

    _____True _____False

14. You refuse to be seen in a bathing suit, even if the only one on the beach is you.

    _____True _____False

Scoring Yourself: Give yourself two points for each question you answered "False" from questions 1 through 8. If you answered "True" to questions 9, 10, 11, and 12, give yourself two points for each. Give yourself two points for each "False" you gave to questions 13 and 14. Add up your score.

28–24 points: Fabulous, darling. Have you read this book before?

22–18 points: I'm glad you're here. You need me.

16 and under: We need each other. I've been there, too, and believe me, this is the right program for you.

I'm going to break it to you gently now. It's time to get yourself together. You're the one who lives in that body of yours and you're going to have to make

some time to take care of it. It is a matter of life or death. When somebody tells me they find exercising boring, I respond with my opinion that fat hips, a "spare tire" waistline, and flab are certainly not exciting. Exercise can't be as boring as sitting in a chair, unable to get up because of being too fat. Let's stop making excuses now, and make up a schedule that will exercise a priority in our day's activity.

What Time of Day Is Best to Exercise?

I like to exercise first thing in the morning. I usually get up and get into my running clothes and after a good warm-up, I go outside and run and then do my cool-down, all lasting from forty minutes to an hour or more, depending on how far I run. I usually run a minimum of two miles, six days a week. Vital to my running, however, is my spiritual warm-up.

I also like to do a workout in the early evening because I have a tendency to eat at night. It's no problem for me to go without breakfast and lunch but when dinner comes I can become a wild Godzilla in the kitchen, devouring everything but the handles on the cupboards and the faucets on the sink. I find if I put on my tights and leotards, I will be thinking of Blessercize rather than food.

You may not exercise as long or as frequently as I do, but you will want to set aside a time every single day when you will work out. At the Christian Center for Counseling and Fitness in San Diego, we have aerobics classes beginning at 7:00 A.M. The girls in this class are particularly dedicated to shaping up for the glory of the Lord because it requires extra effort to get up earlier in the morning to exercise.

Types of Exercises That Give Your Body Best Results

There are many exercises which do not show any appreciable effect on your body. The reason for this is either the exercise is aimed only at the skeletal muscles and makes no demands on your lungs, heart, and blood system, or the exercise is done for such a short amount of time that your organs never reach a steady state of exertion where benefits begin.

The five basic exercise categories are:

Isometrics

These exercises involve contracting a muscle without producing movement. For example, you place your palms on either side of your doorway and press for a few seconds. A measurable fitness condition cannot be achieved from exercising only seconds a day in this way, although it helps strengthen muscles.

Isometric exercises can increase the size and strength of your skeletal muscles, but they will not affect your overall health, particularly your pulmonary and cardiovascular systems. If you press against a wall with your arms for ten seconds a day, your muscles will become stronger, but only during that specific activity.

Isometric exercises are good for bed-ridden patients, or when you are sitting for long periods of time, but isometrics work on only one muscle group at a time, and it would take a long time to use all of your muscles. These exercises do not demand enough oxygen and can actually make a joint more vulnerable to injury. Dr. Kenneth Cooper says, "The value of isometrics is to develop muscles to do isometrics . . . and little else."

Isotonics

Isotonic means "equal tension." Examples of isotonic exercises are calis-thenics and weight lifting. These exercises are good for your body, but they are not enough by themselves to produce optimum physical fitness. Calisthenics should not be considered the foundation of any exercise program. They will develop your muscles, slim you down, and build you up, but they will not affect your heart and lungs adequately. That is why the program you are about to engage in includes isotonics as well as the other exercises, including aerobics. Isotonics are basically muscle exercises, and work to strengthen and tone your muscles.

Weight training will increase your muscular strength and endurance, as well as improve your flexibility. Many women are discovering the benefits of working out with weights.

Isokinetics

These exercises are the ones performed on machines. The best-known isokinetic machine is the Nautilus. It's a brand name for weight-lifting machines that allow a muscle group to meet resistance through movement. You lie on a bench or sit on a seat and move weights attached to pulleys and rotary cams. The Universal Machine is another brand name, and offers stations at which you can work twelve different muscle groups. Up to eight people can work out on one machine at a time, going from station to station. The only way to use these machines is to join a health club.

Anaerobics

These exercises are ones that do not give your body enough oxygen. In fact, the term *anaerobics* literally means "without oxygen." The exercise demands oxygen but then ends quickly, such as running frantically for a bus. Another type of anaerobic exercise is the one-hundred-yard dash. These exercises rapidly create large oxygen debts but there is no buildup, pace, or cool-down. You want to do exercises that demand oxygen for a steady period of time. Isotonics and aerobics prepare you for anaerobic experiences.

Aerobics

These are the basis of your exercise program. They will produce the "miracles" you are praying for. Aerobic exercises require a great deal of oxygen. They are swimming, running, rowing, cycling, skipping rope, cross-country skiing, and the aerobic exercises outlined in this book. Among them is our favorite, the David Dance.

Aerobic exercise will strengthen your cardiovascular system, lower your resting pulse rate, keep your body-fat percentage at low levels, and burn calories. These exercises cannot be performed at a minimum level of exertion if they are to benefit you fully. Jogging lazily or paddling around in a pool without effort will not give you an optimum pulse rate. To be aerobically fit, you will be doing any daily exercise nonstop for at least fifteen minutes, which maintains your pulse at 80 percent of 200 minus your age for that amount of time. This you work up to, so don't be worried now. Nobody is going to ask you to swim the English channel or jump rope until the cows come home, for the time being.

Pat yourself on the back (if you can't reach it, have someone else do it for you). You are going to be in for some benefits you didn't expect.

Bless the Lord, O my soul: and all that is within me, bless his holy name. Bless the Lord, O my soul, and forget not all his benefits.

Psalms 103:1, 2

The Lord has given you many benefits because you belong to Him. He not only forgives your sins but He heals your diseases as well. He redeems your life from destruction. He crowns you with lovingkindness and tender mercies. He will satisfy you with good things and renew your youth like the eagle's (Psalms 103:3–5).

"Who healeth all thy diseases." What diseases and what destruction will be removed from your life from now on? Let's look at some of them.

Physical Problems Exercise Helps

Headache

There are countless studies showing that headaches and tension problems which elevate blood pressure and place huge overloads on your circulatory system can be relieved by exercises.

Isn't that great news? Instead of reaching for the aspirin, reach for your leotard and start your workout.

As you begin exercising, you will feel your body relaxing and tension headaches lifting. The reason for this relief is a result of vasodilatation (enlargement of the blood vessels). The increased size of the blood vessels allows a lowering of blood pressure as well as an increase in the amount of oxygen to the brain. Kiss those aspirin good-bye.

Pain in the neck

(I don't mean your in-laws.) Pinched nerves, thoracic outlet syndrome, and a bunch of other names of disorders fit here, but let me tell you, there's nothing like regular exercise to help the condition. I suffered for years from neck-and-shoulder pain because I spend so many hours of my life hunched over my typewriter and huddled with my nose buried in books. I used to suffer terribly, and for a while I was telling my family, "Don't bother to bury me when I die. Just peel me off my typewriter and mail me fourth class to *Christian Bookseller.*"

Since I've been working out every day,

I have absolutely *no* pain in my neck, back, or shoulders. You'll be given specific exercises for your upper body. Do them faithfully *every* day for best results.

Backaches

There are so many disorders of the spine that I won't pretend to be an expert on them all. You need to know your own body. Be sure your physician gives you the okay to start a physical-fitness regimen if you suffer from any back pain. A common reason for back pain is not using your abdominal muscles. All the weight is on your back, unsupported by muscles.

Poor posture, faulty positions of standing and sitting, improper rising, and unbalanced carrying of heavy loads can contribute to back problems. (Spinal curvatures such as kyphosis, lordosis, and scoliosis need to be specially treated with specific exercises and treatment, not covered here). Chances are, if you have a serious deformity of the spinal column you are already engaged in a program specifically designed for your problem. However, if you are like most of us, your backaches are probably due to poor posture, improper weight distribution, faulty positions of standing and sitting, and lack of muscular support. In studies made, 85 percent of Harvard and Yale freshmen showed posture deformities of a functional type. Schoolchildren showed lateral postural deformities to the extent of 34 to 48 percent. (These figures were cited in Herbert M. Shelton's book *Exercise.*)

Your spinal column is a flexible and flexuous column composed of twenty-four separate bones (vertebrae) and held in position by ligaments, and separated by an elastic cartilaginous cushion which permits movement. You're held upright by several layers of muscle running in all directions, like ropes holding all your vital organs together. (*See* the diagram on page 49 and you'll see what I mean.)

Faulty posture produces stress and strain on your precious spinal column, and it rebels with aches and pains. Arnold D., a student of mine, swears he could hear his back hollering, "Ouch!" in the night. It has been discovered that even functional visceral impairments result from bad posture. Muscular weakness, whether resulting from malnutrition or lack of proper exercise, is an important factor in producing faulty positions of sitting and standing.

Dr. Shelton claims that during periods of rapid growth in children in adolescence, the body structure may grow faster than the muscles, and children are then without sufficient strength to support their bodies properly. Vigorous exercise is essential during these periods to obtain muscular strength and development.

How much more, if you lead a sedentary life, do you need to exercise those muscles of yours to support your body properly! If you sit most of the day you will, among other things, develop abdominal-muscle deterioration unless it is counteracted by appropriate exercise.

Although certain cases of faulty posture are beyond your control, most cases are preventable and remediable. Good posture in the lower back depends as much upon the strength and tone of the abdominal muscles as upon that of the muscles of the spine and thighs.

Take courage! You're about to experience new delights as you learn movements to stretch the muscles and ligaments of your chest anterior, the ligaments and muscles of your lumbar, spine, and buttocks, as well as develop muscles of your upper back, shoulders, and abdomen.

Varicose veins

Do you know that about half the adult population of America has varicose veins? Medical authorities tell us that people with varicose veins have congenitally weak-walled veins, and poor nutrition, toxemia, enervation, pregnancy, and *lack of exercise* are huge contributors to the problem.

Have you ever seen an Olympic champion with varicose veins? Find me one professional athlete with a serious case of varicose veins—I dare you. Energetic use of the muscles and accelerated circulation prevent venous stagnation in the legs and will help remedy the problem. See your doctor if you have varicose veins, but for heaven's sake and yours, too, start your Fun to Be Fit program immediately.

Running, jogging, brisk walking, climbing stairs, and exercises with your feet in the air will all help you. You will be flexing and extending your feet and legs, and doing specific leg exercises to strengthen your muscles, as well as engaging in an aerobics program, all of which will help.

Shaping Your Body

You have the life of God in you and the nature of God in you. Say out loud right now:

I am a new creature in Christ. Old things are passed away, behold all things are become new in me. I am not an old, lazy person. I am a new creature with the life of God in me because I am filled with the Spirit of God.

Not Defiling Yourself

Let's look at the book of Daniel. I want you to see something very important:

And the king spake unto Ashpenaz the master of his eunuchs, that he should bring certain of the children of Israel, and of the king's seed, and of the princes; Children in whom was no blemish, but well favoured, and skilful in all wisdom, and cunning in knowledge, and understanding science, and such as had ability in them to stand in the king's palace, and whom they might teach the learning and the tongue of the Chaldeans. And the king appointed them a daily provision of the king's meat, and of the wine which he drank: so nourishing them three years, that at the end thereof they might stand before the king. Now among these were the children of Judah, Daniel, Hananiah, Mishael, and Azariah: Unto whom the prince of the eunuchs gave names: for he gave unto Daniel the name Belteshazzar; and to Hananiah, of Shadrach; and to Mishael, of Meshach; and to Azariah, of Abed-nego. But Daniel purposed in his heart that he would not defile himself with the portion of the king's meat, nor with the wine which he drank: therefore he requested of the prince of the eunuchs that he might not defile himself. Now God had brought Daniel into favour and tender love with the prince of the eunuchs. And the prince of the eunuchs said unto Daniel, I fear my lord the king, who hath appointed your meat and your drink: for why should he see your faces worse liking than the children which are of your sort? then shall ye make me endanger my head to the king. Then said Daniel to Melzar, whom the prince of the eunuchs had set over Daniel, Hananiah, Mishael, and Azariah, Prove thy servants, I beseech thee, ten days; and let them give us pulse to eat, and water to drink. Then let our countenances be looked upon before thee, and the countenance of the children that eat of the portion of the king's meat: and as thou seest, deal with thy servants. So he consented to them in this matter, and proved them ten days. And at the end of ten days their countenances appeared fairer and fatter in flesh than all the children which did eat the portion of the king's meat. Thus Melzar took away the portion of their meat, and the wine that they should drink; and gave them pulse. As for these four children, God gave them knowledge and skill in all learning and wisdom: and Daniel had understanding in all visions and dreams. Now at the end of the days that the king had said he should bring them in, then the prince of the eunuchs brought them in before Nebuchadnezzar. And the king communed with them; and among them all was found none like Daniel, Hananiah, Mishael, and Azariah: therefore stood they before the king. And in all matters of wisdom and understanding, that the king enquired of them, he found them ten times better than all the magicians and astrologers that were in all his realm.

Daniel 1:3–20

Ten times better, their countenance fairer, fatter (healthier) in flesh, skillful in learning and wisdom! How God blessed them! Daniel did not defile himself and "among them all was found none like Daniel."

God gave Daniel wisdom. You also can have the wisdom of God to make choices that are good. Daniel and his friends had the wisdom to refuse the food of the king and choose the food of *their* King.

You have the nature of God, the life of God, and the wisdom of God in you, but if you do not use or appropriate what God has given you, you can never walk in the true light of 2 Corinthians 5:17: "Therefore if any man be in Christ, he is a new creature...."

You are a new creature (a new person) because the Lord has called you to be His own. But just as there are many carnal Christians in other areas of life, you can be a carnal Christian in the fitness area. Remember, you want to be totally developed, body, soul, and spirit. You are developing your spirit and your mentality. God's wisdom is in you and the life of God is in you. The power of God is in you. Begin to speak to yourself as a person of value. Can you imagine Daniel sitting in his room, complaining miserably that he couldn't eat the king's greasy casseroles? Can you just see Daniel sneaking out of bed at night and heading for the king's kitchen in search

of a prune Danish or a jelly doughnut?

No, it was Daniel's idea to abstain from eating the king's food. Daniel purposed in his heart that he would not defile or hurt himself. Will you purpose in your heart now not to defile yourself? Affirm these powerful truths:

I Will Not Hurt Myself By . . .

- Eating when I am not hungry.
- Eating heavy, fattening food when I am hungry because I must have something *this instant*.
- Spending most of my time sitting, standing, or lying down.
- Spending a lot of money to join a health spa and only showing up five times all year.
- Telling myself that housework or washing the car is all the exercise I need.
- Keeping all the exercise equipment I bought to get in shape four years ago in the garage, covered with dust.
- Hiding out at home and not going places because I'm embarrassed about my physical appearance.
- Never wearing fitted clothes in order to hide the flab.
- Living in a constant state of lethargy and overall weariness.
- Telling myself I'm too fat to exercise. (That is just not true. Start slowly after checking with your doctor, and you'll do great.)
- Continuing to overeat when exercising. (The Lord is right at your side, ready to start when you are.)

Dear Lord, I have given You the right to be Lord of my body, and now I need to know how very close You are to me as I start my new fitness program. I know it is an entire new way of life, and I accept that. I choose to be healthy and fit for Your sake, and I dedicate myself to being fit and in shape for the rest of my life. I refuse to consider this a crash program because my body is too precious to crash.

I now purpose in my heart, as Daniel did, not to defile or hurt myself. I will not hurt myself with slothful life habits of any kind. I am a new creature daily in You. My old, lazy habits are a thing of the past. I love You, Jesus, Lord of my muscles and bones, as well as my soul and spirit. I know You love all of me.

_____

(Your Name)

Don't you feel better already? Of course you do. You're committed to God, ready to experience His power in your life in a new way; you're determined to conquer old habits. Onward and upward then with the program. Your program is in four parts:

I. Warm-up
II. Stretching and Calisthenics
(specific parts of the body worked out)
III. Aerobics
IV. Cool-down

The Importance of the Warm-up and Cool-down

I can't stress these two parts of your program enough. They are as important as your breathing. Not long ago, a man came to me complaining of terrible pain in his joints and knees. His running program didn't seem to be that strenuous to warrant such pain. When I questioned him about a warm-up and cool-down, he wasn't sure what I was talking about. As soon as he began adding an adequate warm-up and cool-down exercise time to his running program, the aches and pains in his legs disappeared. If you are planning on running, you will certainly want to warm up and cool down to avoid shinsplints and other injuries.

Warming up includes stretching and getting your pulse rate up. Your metabolic system will get itself ready for the exercises to come at this time. The blood vessels in your muscles will expand and get themselves ready for your time of exercise. If a cold, tight muscle is suddenly shocked into violent contraction such as fast running with no warm-up, it can tear, pull, or strain. An injury can occur in a muscle fascia (the sheath covering the muscle) or in a tendon, ligament, cartilege, or even in a bone in the form of a stress fracture. I'm telling you all of this to emphasize the importance of lengthening and warming your muscle fibers so they can accommodate the strain of exercise.

A gradual toning or conditioning of your muscles will occur as you stretch and contract. You will be exercising each isolated group of muscles as you proceed through your program, moving from your head to your shoulders, to your arms and hands, to your rib cage, waist, hips, spine, buttocks, thighs, lower legs, and feet in a logical progression. Relax and stretch easily, breathing slowly and rhythmically in your warm-up.

You will be warming up in another way, too. This is perhaps the most important warm-up of all, because it is the very heart and core of your entire fitness program. This warm-up is your *spiritual* warm-up. It is when you take one Scripture verse and speak it out loud as you stretch. For example, 2 Samuel 22:40: "For thou hast girded me with strength. . . ."

Speak these words out loud. Hear them and believe them. As you start your exercises unto the Lord, you are blessing not only your body but your soul and spirit as well. Continue to repeat your verse throughout your entire warm-up. There is a strong principle I am stressing here, and it is the principle of scriptural meditation. Joshua 1:8 reads:

This book of the law shall not depart out of thy mouth; but thou shalt meditate therein day and night, that thou mayest observe to do according to all that is written therein: for then thou shalt make thy way prosperous, and then thou shalt have good success.

You are meditating on the Word of God as you speak it to yourself over and over again. You will find yourself becoming as strong as you tell yourself you are, not only physically but in every single area of your life. That's why I call our workouts "Blessercize."

Scripture Verses to Meditate On as You Exercise

Notice I make God's powerful promises personal. Get *involved* with God's Word. Get intimate with His Word. Make it live in your heart, like fire. You do this by speaking it to yourself, meditating on what you're saying, and allowing the Holy Spirit to kindle life and power within you. It cannot fail to make a dynamic impact on your life.

God instructs me and teaches me the way I should go. He councils me with His eye upon me.

See Psalms 32:8, 9

Nothing separates me from the love of Christ. Not tribulation, distress, persecution, famine, nakedness, peril or sword.

See Romans 8:35–39

This I know, that thou art pleased with me.

See Psalms 41:11

I am strong and of good courage. I am not frightened or dismayed, for the Lord, my God, is with me wherever I go.

See Joshua 1:9

When I pass through the waters the Lord is with me; and through the rivers, they shall not overflow me: when I walk through the fire, I shall not be burned, neither shall the flames kindle upon me.

See Isaiah 43:2

I will not let my heart be troubled. I believe in God and I believe in the Lord Jesus Christ. In my Father's house are many mansions: if it were not so, the Lord would have told me.

See John 14:1, 2

All things are possible to me because I believe.

See Mark 9:23

I submit myself to God. I resist the devil and he flees from me.

See James 4:7

Part II of your exercise program is your specific body-shaping exercises. During these exercises you will count and speak the Word to yourself at the same time. We use only Christian music on the Fun to Be Fit program. Records by Dallas Holm, Andrae Crouch, Evie, the 2nd Chapter of Acts, Leon Patillo, the Agape Force, the Rambos, and so many other wonderful Christian artists are fun to exercise by. Find your own favorites. You'll bless your body, soul, and spirit listening to the words of the songs as you exercise.

Part III of your exercise period will be your aerobics. Here's where you let loose and have a ball. It precedes the best part of all, the David Dance. Then the fourth and final phase is your cool-down period. The cool-down consists of basically the same stretches you warmed up with. The purpose of the cool-down is to allow your pulse rate to return to normal. *Never* stop exercises abruptly. Always walk at least five minutes after you have finished running or any of the aerobic activities on the chart on page 64. After your exercise program, your cool-down exercises will complete your daily exercise routine. The cool-down will help prevent sore muscles and bring your entire system back to normal.

Now let's get on with the program itself. Let's start by taking some nice, deep breaths. Inhale through your nose and hold your breath for the count of six. Now very evenly let the air out while holding your stomach in and your back straight. Blow out through your mouth. Do this exercise three times. You will find if you do this exercise throughout the day, your sinus problems, headaches, and tense upper-body muscles will feel a lot better. Now we are ready for our warm-up.

The Spirit of the Lord God is upon me; because the Lord hath anointed me to preach good tidings unto the meek; he hath sent me to bind up the brokenhearted, to proclaim liberty to the captives, and the opening of the prison to them that are bound; To proclaim the acceptable year of the Lord, and the day of vengeance of our God; to comfort all that mourn; To appoint unto them that mourn in Zion, to give unto them beauty for ashes, the oil of joy for mourning, the garment of praise for the spirit of heaviness; that they might be called trees of righteousness, the planting of the Lord, that he might be glorified.

Isaiah 61:1-3

THE EXERCISE PROGRAM

PART I
THE WARM-UP

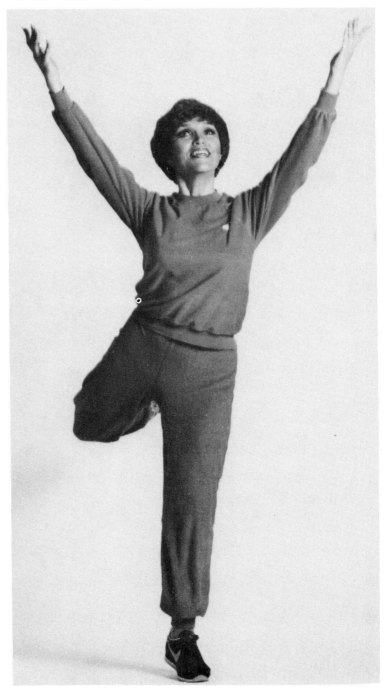

1 Head Rolls

Stand up real straight, shoulders and arms relaxed, stomach in, buttocks tucked under, feet about 18 inches apart.

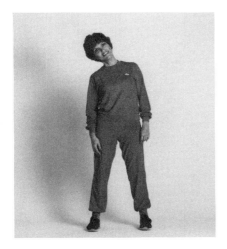

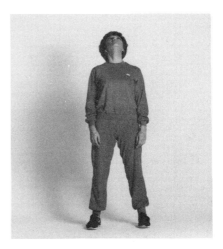

1. Drop your head right to the side for 1 count. Feel the stretch up the left side of your neck.

2. Now roll your head to the back, chin to the ceiling, for 1 count. Let your mouth hang open.

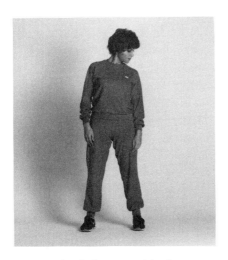

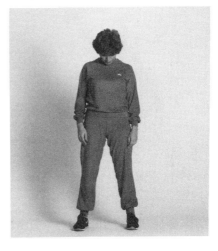

3. Rotate to the left smoothly for a count of 1, with your ear parallel to your shoulder.

4. Continuing the movement, drop your head forward, chin to chest.

Repeat the series 3 times to the right and 3 times to the left.

If your neck creaks and cracks while doing this exercise, it shows your need for it.

79

2 Shoulder Circles

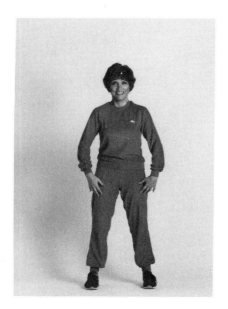 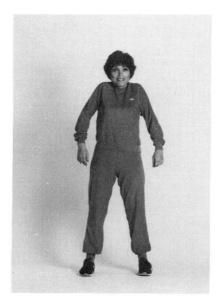

1. Standing erect, push your shoulders forward to a count of 1. Keep your neck relaxed.

2. Lift shoulders up toward the ceiling to the count of 1.

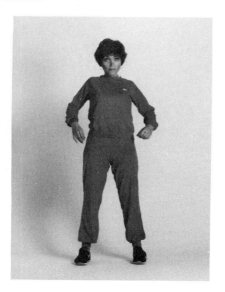 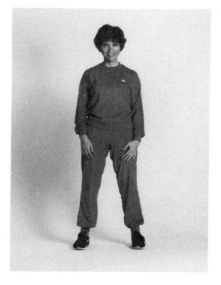

3. Push shoulders gently back, but hard, to the count of 1.

4. Drop them down and repeat.

Repeat circles 3 times to the front and 3 times to the back. Work up to 6. Do these exercises during the day to get rid of stiff neck and shoulders.

3 Jacob's Ladder

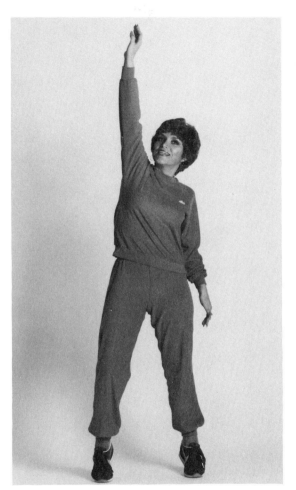 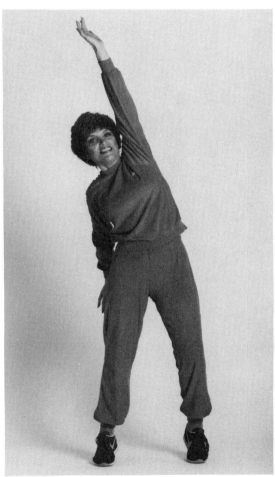

Standing with feet 8 inches apart, lift your arms and reach first with the right and then with the left arm over your head. Raising up on your toes, feel as though you're being held erect by an invisible string pulling you up by the head. Don't hunch those shoulders.

20 reaches
10 each arm
breathe evenly

4 Side Bends

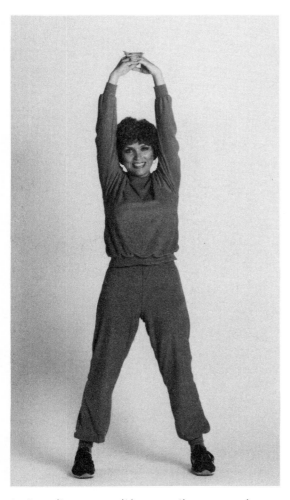 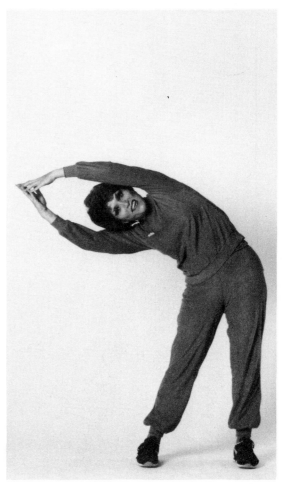

1. Standing erect, lift your rib cage and clasp hands in front of you. Raise your hands over your head and stretch.

20 side bends
10 to left
10 to right

2. Bend straight to the right side. Feel that wonderful pull along your waist and left side. Count to 2. Repeat on other side.

5 Hamstring and Vertebrae Stretches

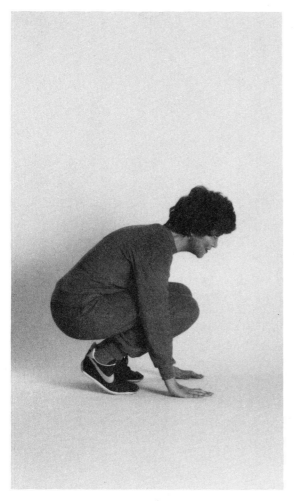

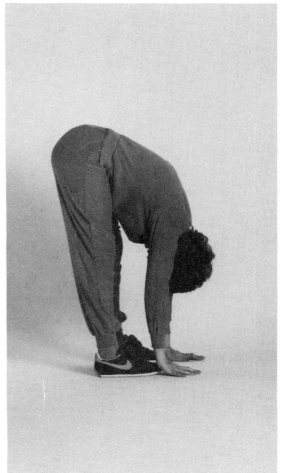

1. Feet together, bend knees and place hands flat on floor.

2. Straighten knees, keeping your head tucked under. Keep your palms flat on the floor.

Do this 6 times.

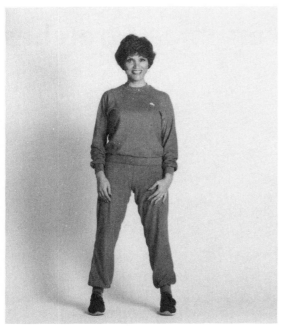

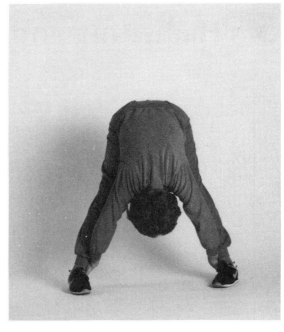

1. Spread feet apart, toes slightly in.

2. Slowly lower your torso until your hands reach your feet. Grab both ankles so your head pokes between your knees. Pull on your ankles to stretch as far as you can. Don't bounce!

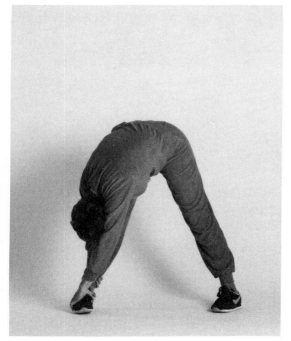

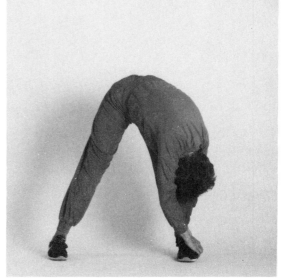

3. Now put your torso over your right leg. Count to 4 as you bring head to right knee.

4. Pull torso over your left leg. Count to 4.

Roll up and slowly repeat. Do this 4 more times and work up to 8 or more.

6 Tendon Stretch

To strengthen calf muscles.

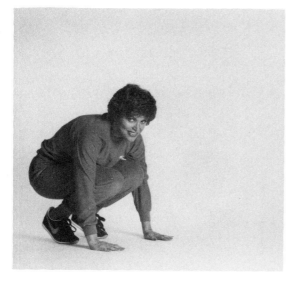

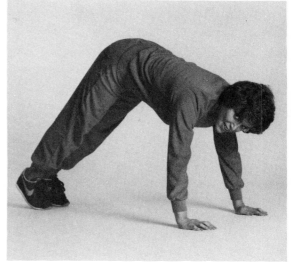

1. Start in bent-knee position with palms flat on floor and head loose. Feet are 18 inches apart.

2. Slowly walk your hands away from your body.

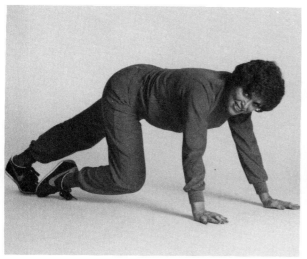

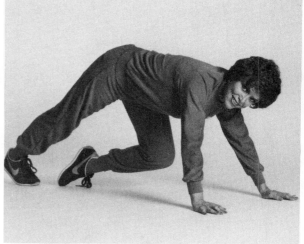

3. Lift your heels off the floor and straighten your knees. With your left heel up, bend your right knee to stretch. Hold for 4 counts.

Do 4 times on each side.

4. Repeat the same on other side.

/ **Lunge and Stretch**

Add this exercise after two weeks. Exhale as you stretch over your leg.

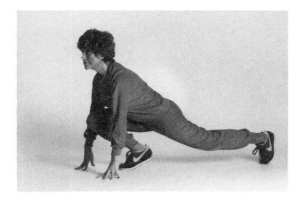

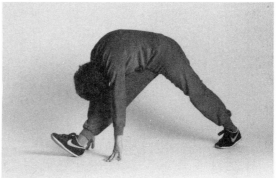

1. Lunge forward on right foot with left leg stretched out behind you. Hand brace yourself on floor.

2. Distribute your weight so you can straighten front leg while flexing foot. Pull your head to your knee.

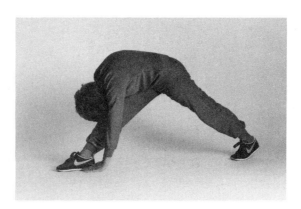

3. Place front foot flat and stretch your torso down farther. Isn't this *fun?*

Do this 10 times on each side and work up to 20.

86

8 Straddle Stretch

Terrific for legs, waist, inner and outer thighs, and buttocks.

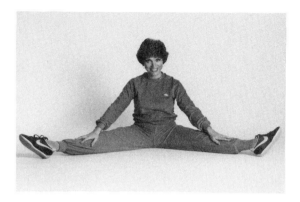

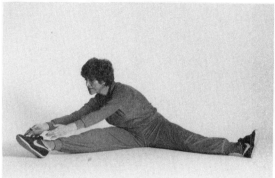

1. Sit on floor with legs stretched as wide as possible. Point your toes. Don't worry if your legs make a narrow V, you'll get better as your tendons stretch.

2. Turn to the right and stretch over the right leg with your chest aimed at your knee, to the count of 4.

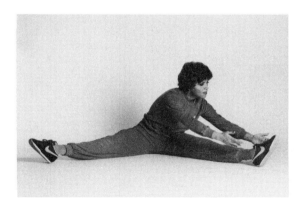

3. Keeping your body low, swing to the left and stretch over your left leg, to the count of 4.

Repeat 10 times each side. Add arms over head and stretch to each side, 10 times each side.

Add side elbow bends. Put arms behind head with elbows pointed out. Now bend your torso over so elbow touches right knee. Straighten. Now bend to the left so elbow reaches over left knee.

10 times each side.

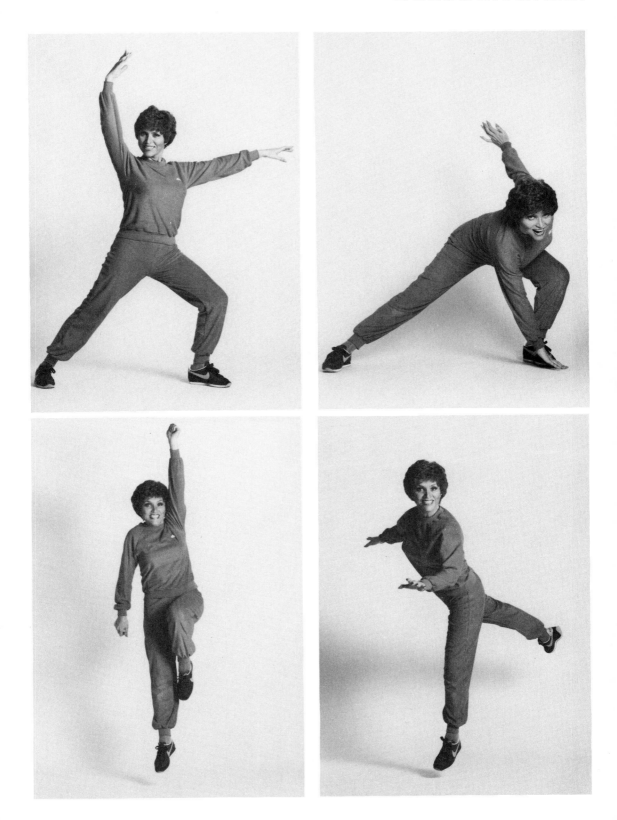

Thighs, Legs, and Hips

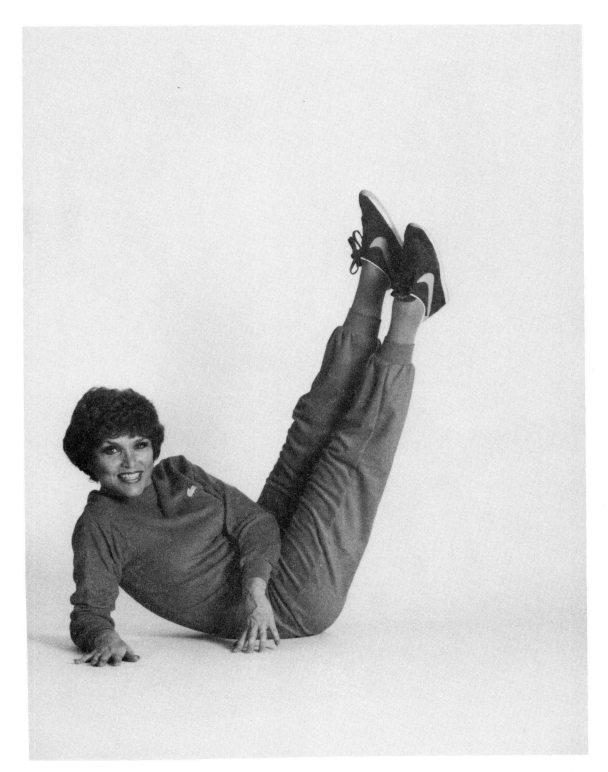

1 Baalam's Donkey Kicks

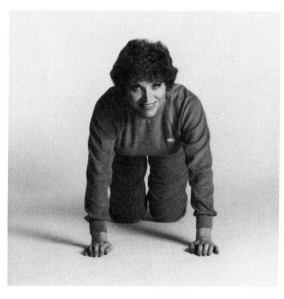

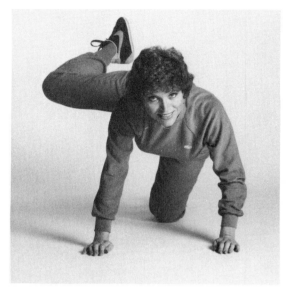

1. Begin on hands and knees with a flat back and head up.

2. Lift right knee out to the side, thigh parallel to floor.

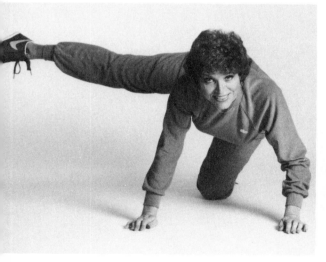

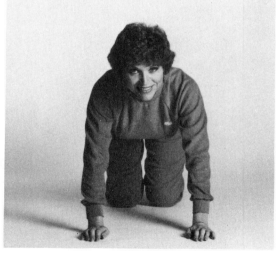

3. Straighten leg with flexed foot.

4. Bring knee back to starting position, but don't let it rest on floor.

Repeat 10 times on each side. Work up to 25 gradually. Increase to 50. This exercise works for the gluteus maximus, medius, minimus, tensor fasciae latae, and sartorius—in other words, where you need it most.

2 Arabesque Kicks

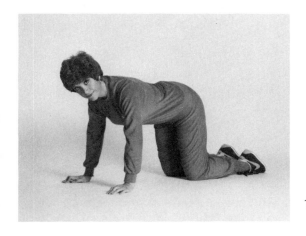

1. Begin on hands and knees with a flat back and head up.

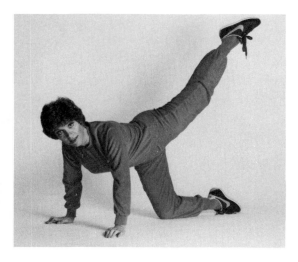

2. Kick leg as high as you can behind you, keeping knee straight. Do these quickly, up-down, up-down.

Do 25 times, increasing to 50 times.

3 Bent-Knee Kicks

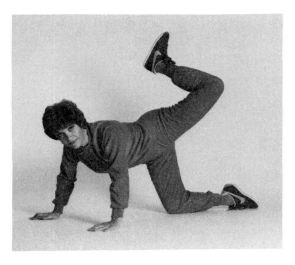

1. Still in Arabesque position, bend knee and flex foot.

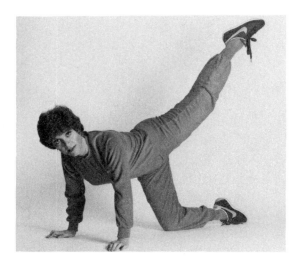

2. Kick and extend knee back. Don't let head fall or back slump.

Repeat 10 times and gradually increase to 25.

4 Thigh Lifts

These are good for your inner thighs. Good-bye, cellulite (water and toxin-logged fat cells)!

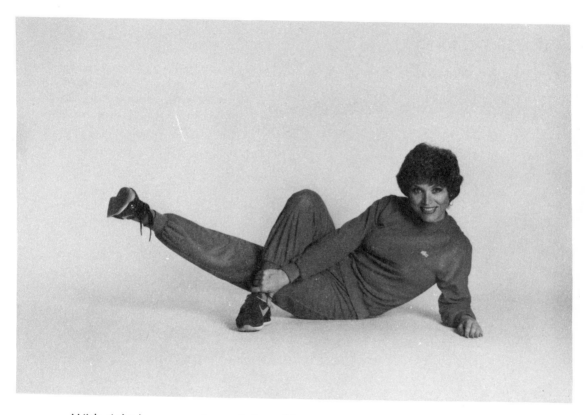

With right leg crossed over left and held by your right hand, lift your left leg as high as you can without bending knee. Keep it straight and lower it. Repeat 10 times, up and down, working up to 50 times on each side.

5 Side Leg Lifts

You'll firm up quickly with this one.

Lift each leg up and down from 3 positions.

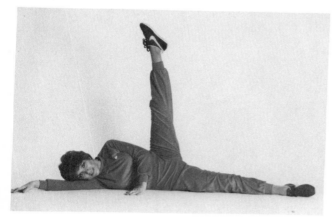

First position: Lie on your right side on the floor with your head resting on your supporting arm. Raise left leg as high as possible and lower it (10 times).

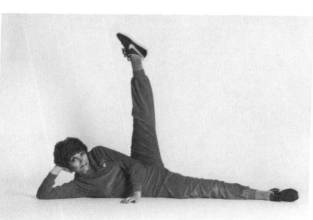

Second position: Rest weight on right elbow.

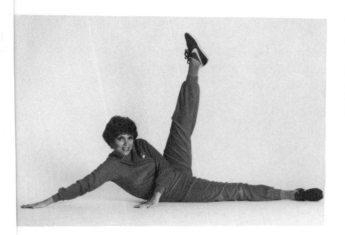

Third position: Straighten supporting arm. Use those stomach muscles.

Do the side leg lift 10 times with pointed foot and 10 times with flexed foot, totaling 30 on each side. You may gradually increase.

6 Scissor Lift

You'll love this one. So will your thighs.

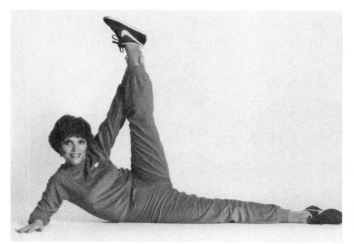

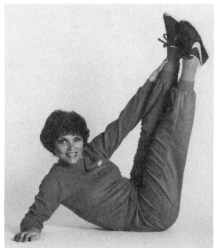

1. Sit on right buttock and rest on your elbow. Hold the ankle of your left leg, keeping that leg as straight as possible.

2. Lift your other leg to meet it. Then lower and repeat. Do this 10 times. Then do it without holding your ankle, like this:

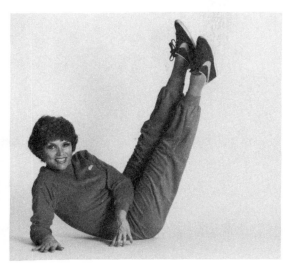

3. An easier version with both arms in front of you: Counting 1-2-3-4, lift left leg. Bring other leg up to meet it. Lower right leg, lower left leg. Repeat on both sides 10 times.

Enjoy these motions. Tell your body to have fun. Think, *Hips, loosen up; fat, go away; muscles, be strong for Jesus.*

"I can do all things through Christ who strengthens me" (*see* Philippians 4:13).

7 Slim and Firm

For a drooping backside.

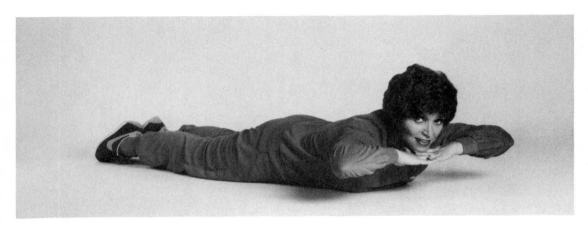

1. Lie on stomach with legs straight and feet together. Rest hands under either chin or hips.

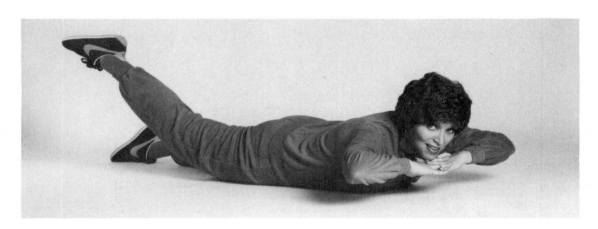

2. Lift right leg high off floor with pointed toe. Hold. Lower leg to floor. Lift left leg high off floor, hold, and lower.

Repeat and add flexed toe when foot is in the air. Alternate leg 10 times; work gradually to 20.

8 Stretch Out

Prayer position.

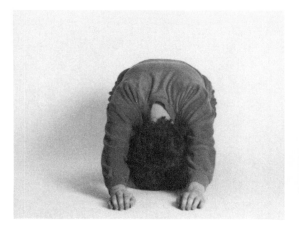

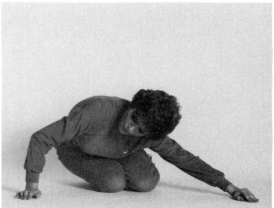

1. *Thank You, Jesus.* Sit back on your heels. Round your body over your knees and reach your arms as far as you can in front of you. Hold for a count of 10.

2. Now move your hips from side to side slowly to stretch the gluteus maximus, first to the right. . .

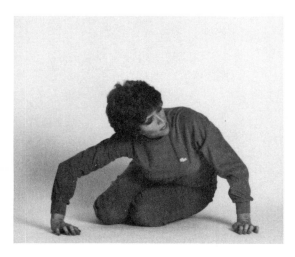

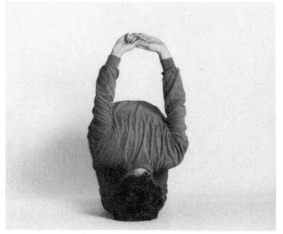

3. . . . and to the left. Relax and thank God for your muscles.

4. Now clasp your hands behind you, and with straight arms, lift them as high as you can. Repeat this final stretch 4 times.

If you must stop between exercises, do not allow more than one minute to elapse. Keep moving.

Never sit and relax between exercises.

Flow from one set to another to work all the muscle groups most effectively and keep up your heart rate.

Stomach, Midriff, and Abdominals

To develop strong muscles, increase circulation, and burn up excess stored fat.

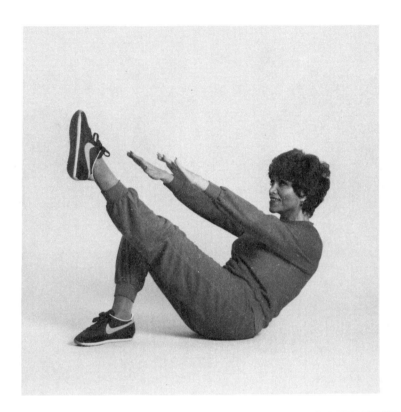

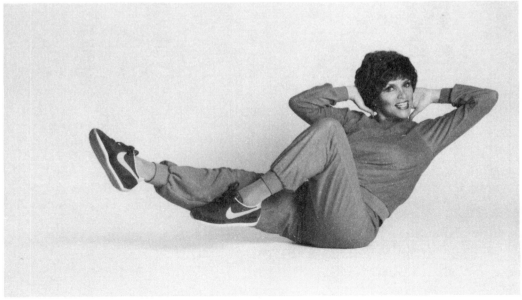

1 Mini Sit-ups

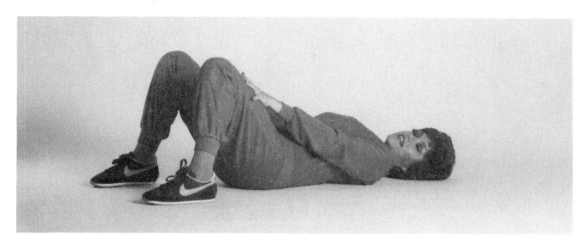

1. Lie on your back, knees bent, feet flat on floor with feet and knees parallel, about 12 inches apart. Place hands on thighs.

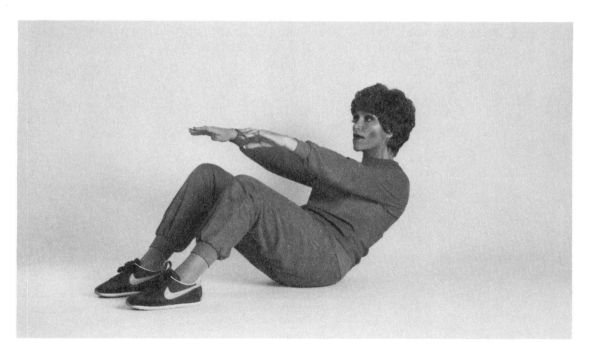

2. Lift your head and upper back off floor, reaching forward. Use your abdominal muscles. Lower your body but do not let your head touch the floor.

Repeat 5 times, increase to 20.
Breathing: Exhale as you lift your body, inhale as you lower it.

101

2   The Bicycle

This will get rid of that "spare tire" stomach.

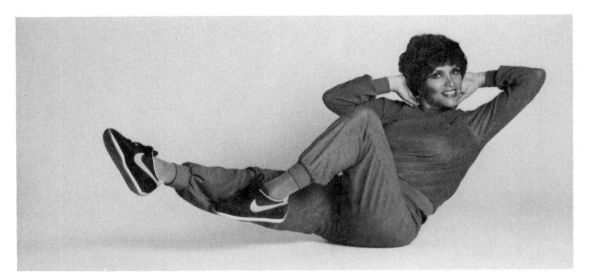

1. Place your hands behind your head and extend your right leg straight out, a few inches off the floor. Point your toe. Bend your left knee to your chest. Reach your elbow to touch your left knee.

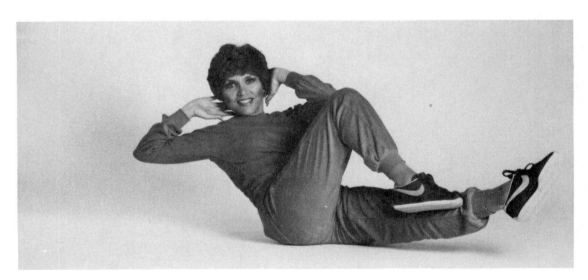

2. Do the same on the other side, extending the left leg out. Keep your toes pointed. Bend your right knee and touch your left elbow to it.

Repeat these movements in a bicycle-peddling motion for a total of 10 counts. Repeat the exercise 10 times with feet flexed. Breathe steadily.

3 Bless Your Stomach

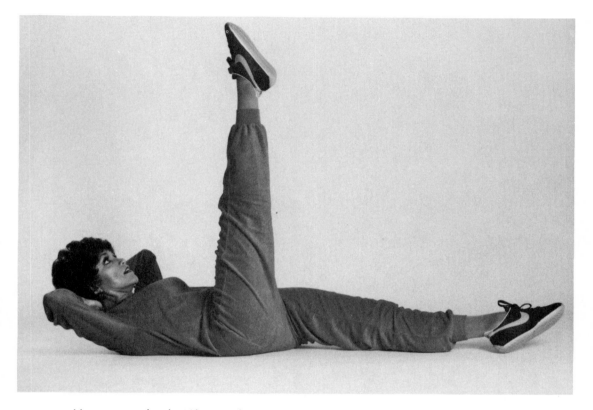

Lie on your back. Lift your head and hold with hands. Raise your leg slowly. Lower it. Now raise your left leg and lower it. Increase speed. Hold that stomach in! You're doing well. Repeat 20 times.

4 Flutter Kicks

To tighten and strengthen abdominal muscles. Eliminates the "spare tire."

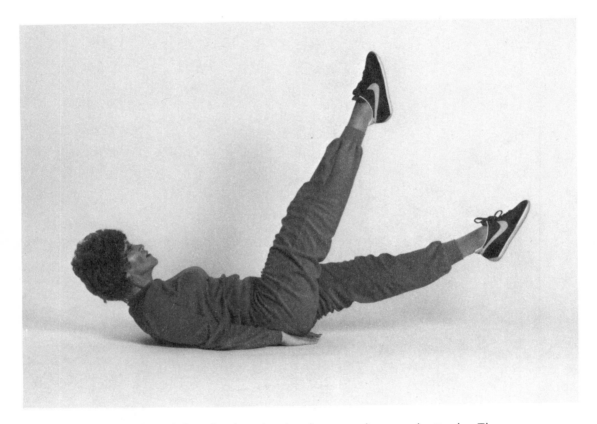

Lie on back with hands placed palm down under your buttocks. The small of the back should touch the floor throughout the exercise. Raise your head and extend and raise your legs. Alternately flex and extend each leg from the hip, but do not touch the floor. Count to 10 while flutter kicking, or recite Micah 6:8. Repeat.

5 Jackknives

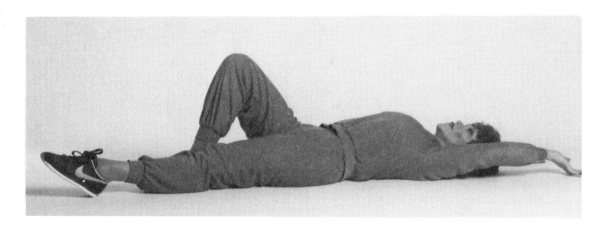

1. Lying flat on the floor with hands and arms over head, bend right knee, keeping left leg straight.

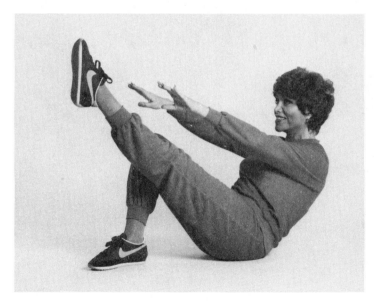

2. Now lift your upper body as your left leg lifts at the same time. Lower and repeat.

Do this exercise 5 times on each side. Then increase to 10 times on each side.

Be sure to hold your stomach tight as you do this exercise. Use your muscles. Breathe in as you relax and breathe out as you lift your body up. This will firm you quickly.

Arms and Chest

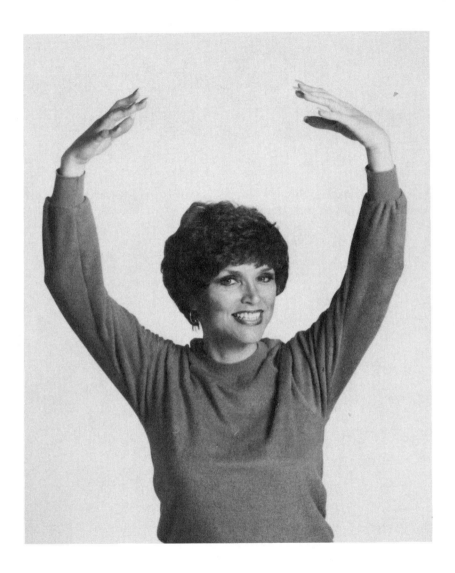

1 Arm Circles

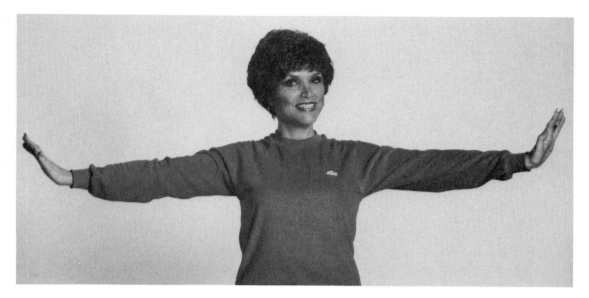

1. Stand erect, stomach in, feet together, and position arms straight out. Now make tiny circles forward with arms as fast as you can.

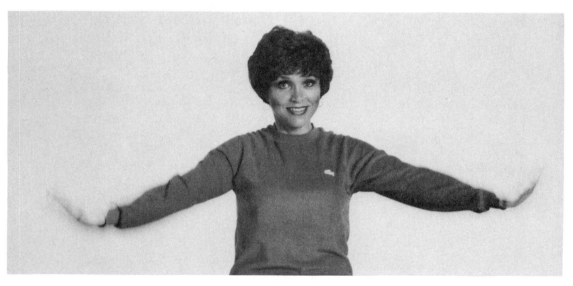

2. Repeat 15 times clockwise and 15 times counterclockwise.

2 Chest and Shoulder Strengthener

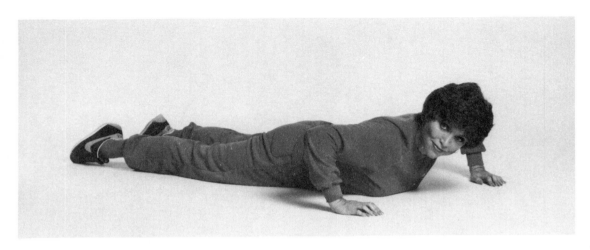

1. Lie facedown on floor with your legs together and toes pointed. Place your arms directly under your shoulders, with your elbows bent and palms flat on floor.

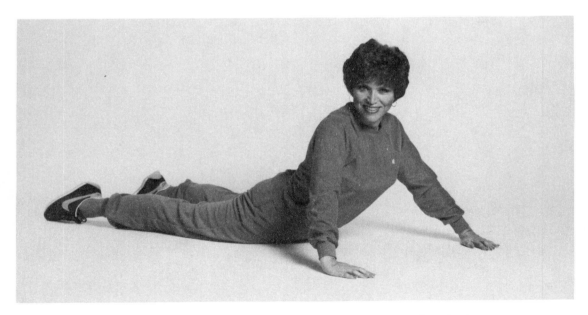

2. Slowly raise the front part *only* off the floor. Lift your head, chest, stomach, and hips up until your arms are straight. Hold. Keep your back straight. Slowly return to starting position.

Repeat 4 times and increase gradually to 12.

3 Mini Push-ups

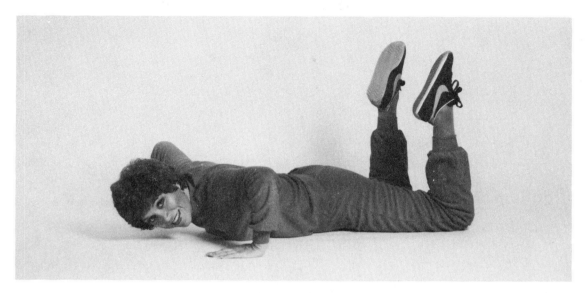

1. Lying on stomach with elbows out and palms flat, bend your knees behind you and point toes.

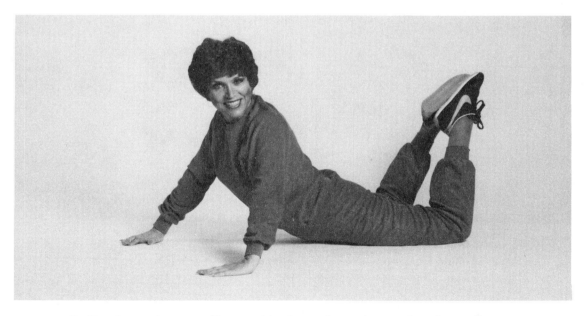

2. Slowly push yourself up with the palms of your hands until your elbows are straight. Now lower your upper body until your chin touches the floor. Repeat.

Do these 5 times to begin with, and work up to 20.

4 Elbow Circles

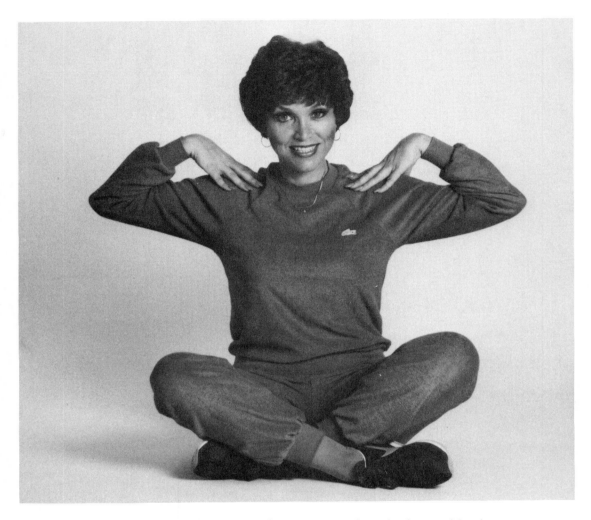

Sit cross-legged on the floor with your stomach tucked in and back straight. Place your hands on your shoulders with fingers pointed. Rotate both elbows in a circle. Begin by lowering elbows down to the side, touching waist. Then point your elbows forward and up, back, and to shoulder level again. Make big circles in the air to begin with and then smaller ones. Repeat 4 circles forward and 4 backward. Increase gradually to 10 in each direction.

When doing your arm and shoulder exercises, try not to move any other part of your body. The muscles in the under and back parts of your arm are generally inactive. These exercises will tone and strengthen those muscles, as well as get rid of flab. Your chest and pectoral muscles will be strengthened and firmed as well.

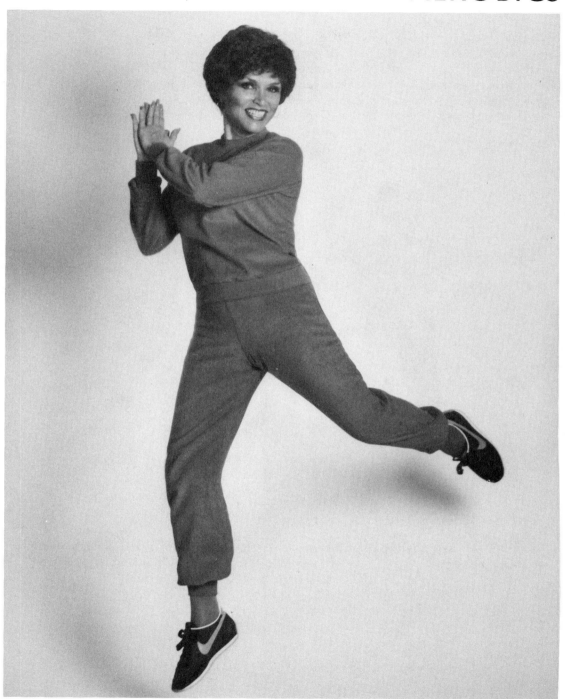

Whatever you do, do your work heartily, as for the Lord rather than for men; knowing that from the Lord you will receive the reward of the inheritance. It is the Lord Christ whom you serve.

Colossians 3:23, 24 NASB

1 Aerobics

You are going to move now, using the muscles you have already warmed up and exercised. The following movements are to be done with slight jumping motions. Jump those inches away. These are joyful and bouncy movements. Put as much energy as you can into these rhythmic, happy exercises. It's like dancing. Suggested music: Dallas Holm, "Hey, I'm a Believer Now," from his album *Dallas Holm and Praise.*

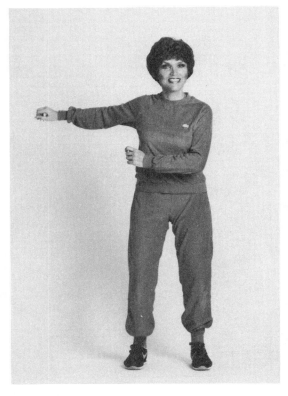

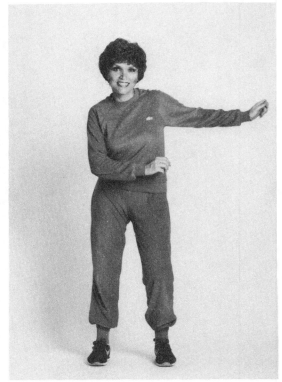

1. Standing with feet slightly apart, begin to rock side to side.

2. Now jump with a bouncy movement side to side. Add a clap by bouncing 1-2-3 clap, 1-2-3 clap.

2 Jog and Jump

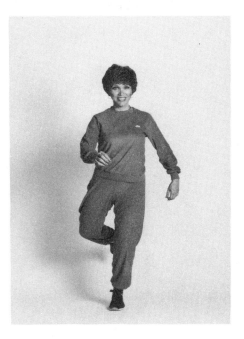

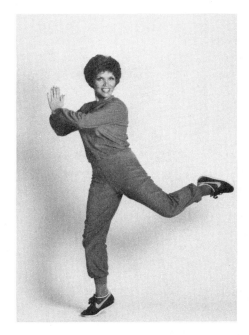

1. Begin with feet together and arms in jogging position. Now jog forward three steps, starting with your right foot.

2. Hop on your right foot, lifting your left knee as high as you can. Clap.

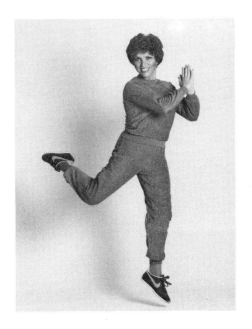

3. Jog back 3 steps, beginning with your left foot. Hop on left foot as you lift your right knee as high as you can. Clap.

Do each exercise 4 times as a set. Then repeat set again.

3 Heel-Toe Jump

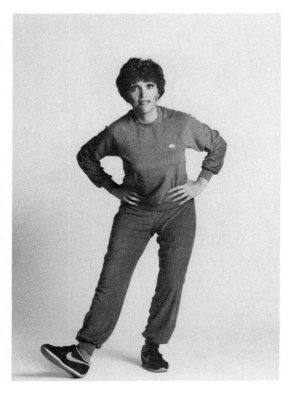 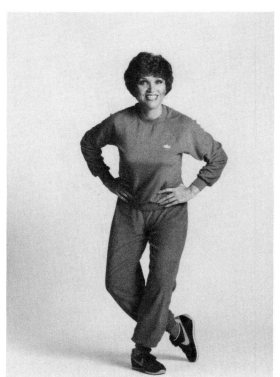

1. Place hands on hips and right heel out to side.

2. Bring heel back in, touch toe to floor, and bring it out again. Do these quickly, out-in, out-in, counting 1-2, 1-2. Repeat on left side.

Do this 8 times on each side.

4 Jump and Praise the Lord

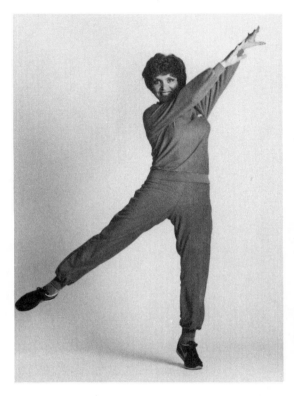

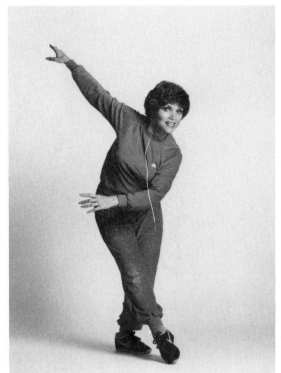

1. Begin with feet together and arms in jogging position. Now as your right foot swings to the side, raise your arms to the ceiling.

2. Now bring your right foot across your left foot and swing your arms across your chest.

Do this 4 times to the right and 4 times to the left. Remember to bounce.

5 Jog in Place

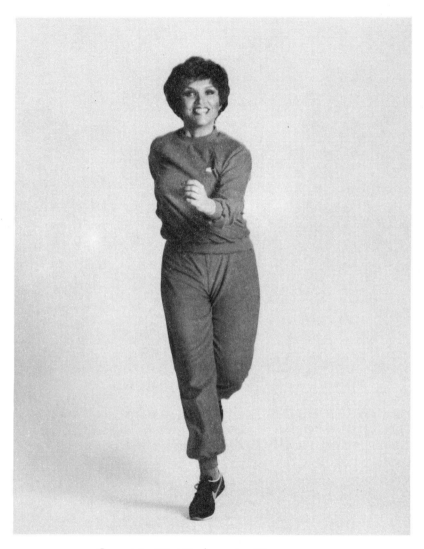

Count to 10. Work up to 60 or more.

6 The Fun Lunge

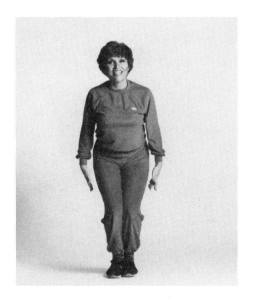

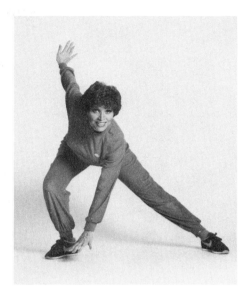

1. Starting in jogging position, jump in place, landing on both feet with knees bent.

2. Now lunge to the right side onto the right foot. Swing your arms in windmill fashion, with your left hand touching the floor.

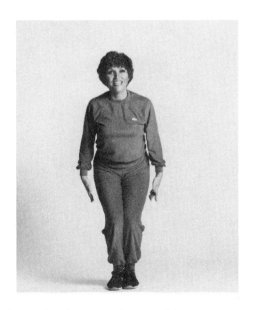

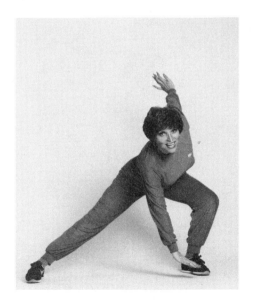

3. Jump back to starting position.

4. Then lunge to the left side.

Do these lunges evenly while holding your stomach muscles in. You will enjoy the stretch you feel in the waist and the inner thigh.

7 The Flick-Flack Kick

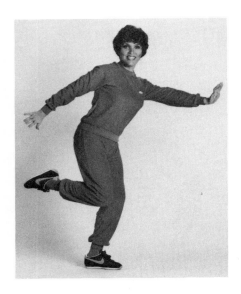

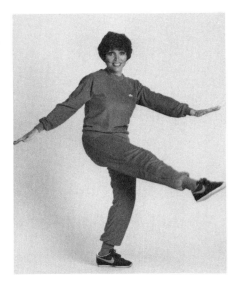

1. With your left knee slightly bent, lift your right foot behind you.

2. Flick and kick your right foot straight forward as you hop lightly on your left foot.

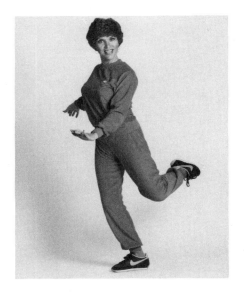

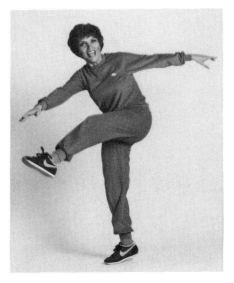

3. Turn and jump onto your right foot as you lift your left foot behind you.

4. Kick your left foot straight forward, and hop lightly on your right foot. Jump onto your left foot as you return to your starting position.

The rhythm is flick-kick, jump, flack-kick, jump. Alternate your feet and enjoy!

8 Forward-Back Jumps

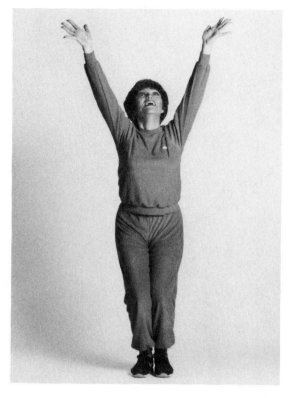

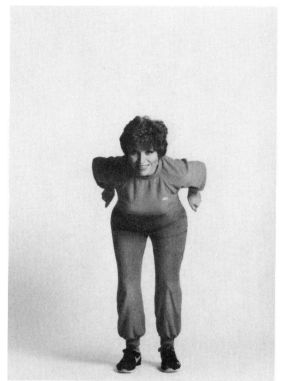

1. Jump forward on both feet with knees slightly bent and arms thrust up and over your head.

2. Jump back on both feet on bent knees, and pull arms back and up behind you.

Repeat this 4 times.

9 Windmill Jumps

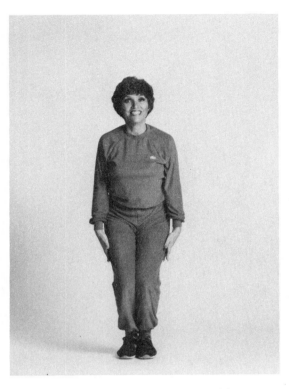

1. Start with knees bent, arms at sides.

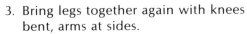

2. Jump out with hands over head and legs apart.

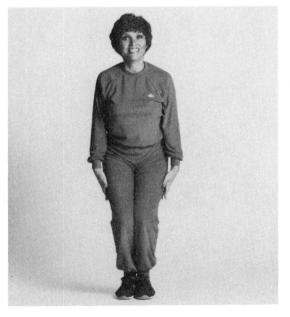

3. Bring legs together again with knees bent, arms at sides.

Do this 8 times.

10 Worship Leaps

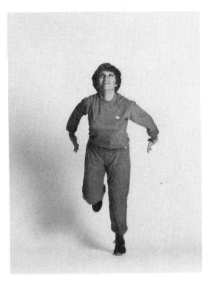

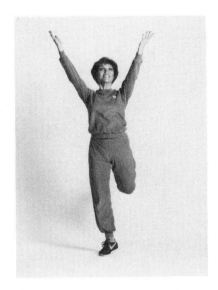

1. Jog in place with hands behind you. Looking up, kick your feet behind you. Count 1-2-3-4.

2. Continue jogging and to the count of 4, raise your arms as high as you can. Leap and whisper, "Praise the Lord."

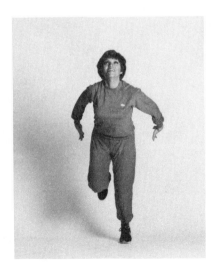

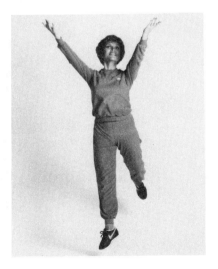

3. Continue jogging and bring arms down to sides to the count of 4. Kick feet behind you.

4. Raise your arms again to the count of 4. Leap and praise the Lord.

You're more than halfway through the entire workout, and so far you are doing beautifully! Stop now, take your pulse, and record it.

To increase your cardiovascular and circulatory strength, repeat the entire aerobics section before going on. You are now ready to go on to the next section, the David Dance.

The David Dance

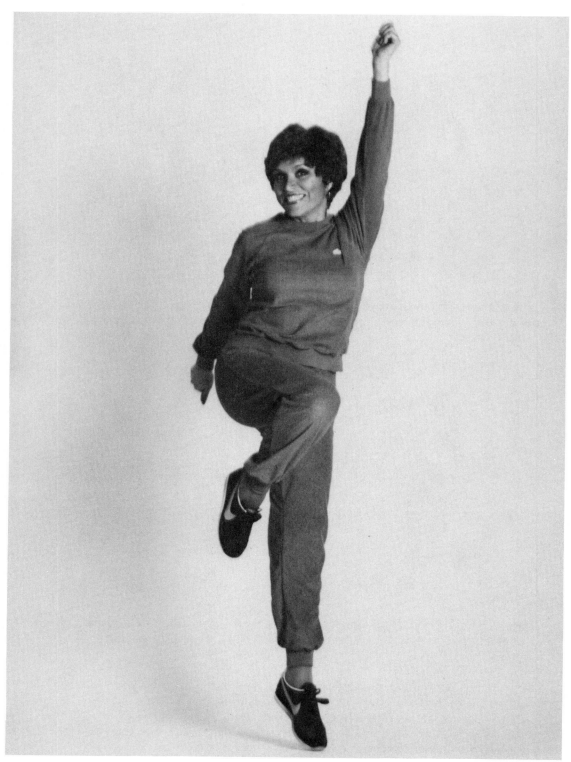

And David danced before the Lord with all
his might. . . ."

2 Samuel 6:14

The David Dance is a celebration of joy and victory, Fun to Be Fit style,
to the Lord. The Bible tells us, "David danced before the Lord with all his
might," when the ark of the covenant was brought into Jerusalem after
having been in the hands of the Philistine enemy.

David danced ecstatically "with all his might," leading a procession of
thirty thousand chosen soldiers and a host of men, women, priests, and
Levites into town with the ark. "Arise, O Lord, into thy rest; thou, and the
ark of thy strength," the royal singers sang (Psalms 132:8). There would be
a tabernacle for the Mighty One of Jacob in Jerusalem!

Unless the Lord shall rest with us there is no rest for us; unless the ark
of His strength live in us we are without strength. Now, nearly three
thousand years later, we can celebrate as David did. We have God resting
within our hearts as the strength of our lives.

Use bouncy, happy music such as I've suggested earlier: Dallas Holm's
"Hey, I'm a Believer Now" or Andrew Culverwell's "Born Again." The
music of Leon Patillo, Evie, Andrae Crouch, the Bill Gaither Trio, plus
scores of others, is also good. Read my instructions carefully and be sure
to note that each segment is repeated several times to the rhythm of the
music. This dance is fun and bright, so let's begin!

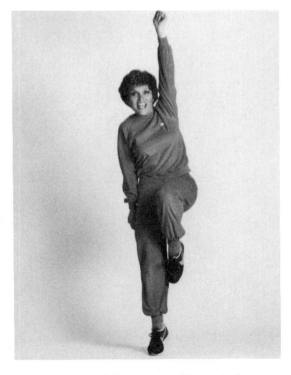 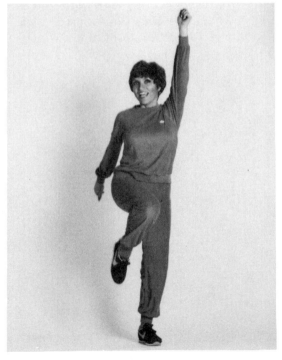

1. Jump onto right foot and hop. Left arm shoots upward.

2. Jump onto left foot and hop. Keep left arm up.

Repeat on opposite side with right arm shooting upward. Do this for 16 counts.

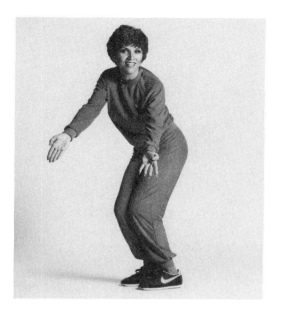 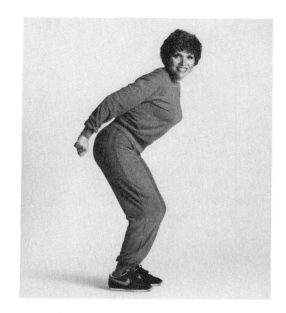

3. Jump to right on both feet with arms straight out, palms open.

4. Jump back, twisting to the left, arms down.

Do this 4 times on the beat for 8 counts. Repeat on the other side, then double time for 8 counts, side to side. Repeat.

5. Jog forward, starting with right foot, slowly raising arms from waist to over your head, to the count of 8.

6. Jog backward, bringing arms down to sides.

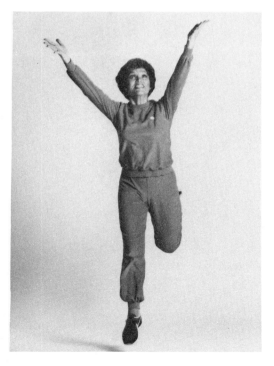 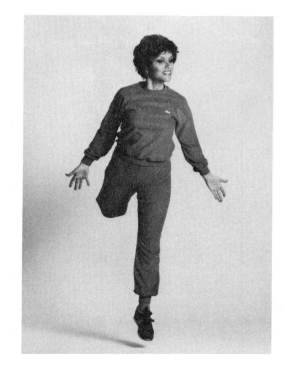

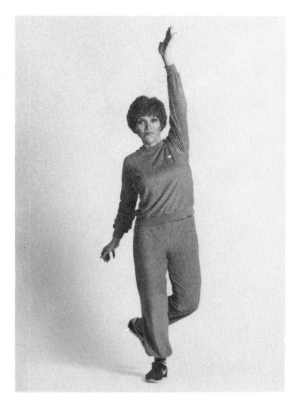 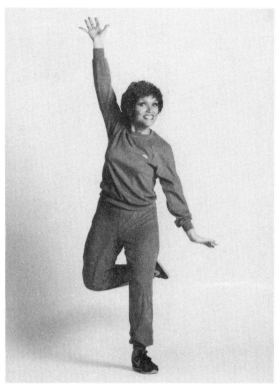

7. a. Hop on right foot, and with quick steps, hop left, right. Then hop on left foot and with quick steps, hop right, left. Rhythm is *right*, left-right. Arms same as step 1.

   b. *Left*, right-left. 16 counts. Repeat jogging step (6) and hop step (7).

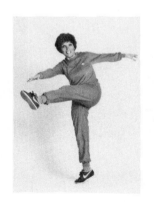 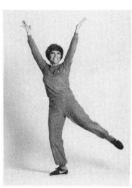 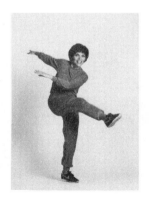 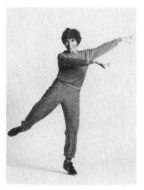

8. a. Jump onto right foot. Hop and kick left foot forward.

   b. Hop and kick left foot back. Repeat for 8 counts.

   c. Reverse the exercise and jump onto left foot, kicking right foot forward.

   d. Hop and kick right foot back. Repeat for 8 counts.

125

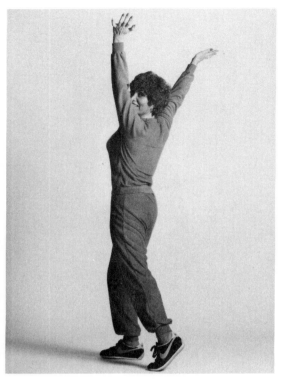 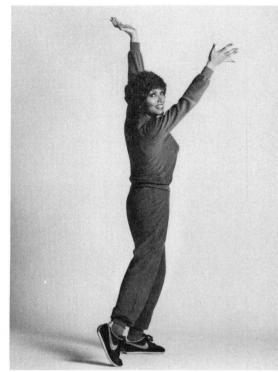

9. Circles:
   a. On right foot, push yourself around in circle to your left with hands over your head for 8 counts, clap on 9th beat.

   b. On left foot, push yourself around in circle to your right with hands over your head. Each circle takes 8 counts, clap on 9th beat.

Do this twice in each direction.

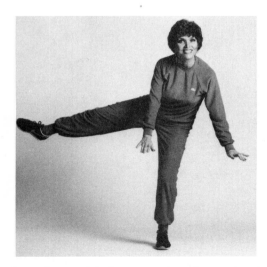 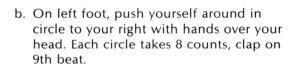 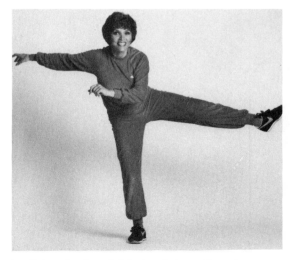

10. a. Start with feet together, knees bent, and kick to the right side.

Repeat for 16 counts.

b. Bring feet quickly back together, knees bent, and kick out to the left side.

126

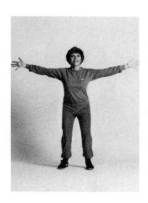 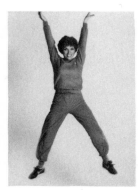 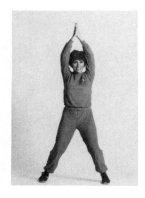 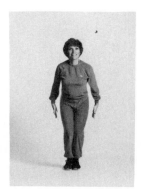

11.a. With arms out to sides, jump on both feet, knees slightly bent.

b. Then leap into the air . . .

c. . . . and land with feet spread apart, as you clap hands together.

d. Return to starting position and repeat sequence.

Do this for 16 counts.

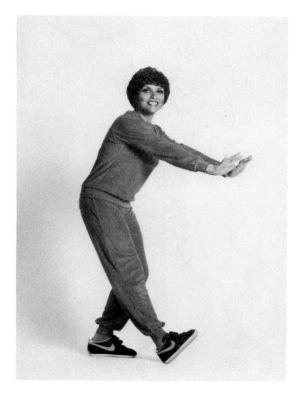 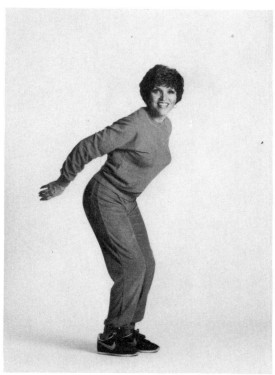

12. a. Turn to your left as you jump onto your left foot, jutting your right foot, heel first, out in front.

b. Then quickly bring your right foot back so your feet are together, arms slightly behind you.

Repeat this sequence quickly 8 times, then switch feet and repeat 8 more times.

127

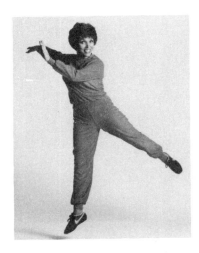 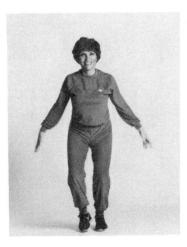 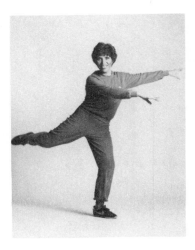

13. a. Lunge to right with arms out . . .

b. . . . then bring feet together . . .

c. . . . and lunge to the left with arms out.

Repeat 8 times on each side.

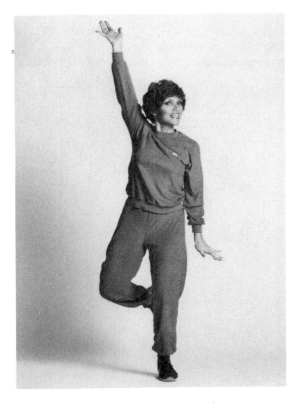 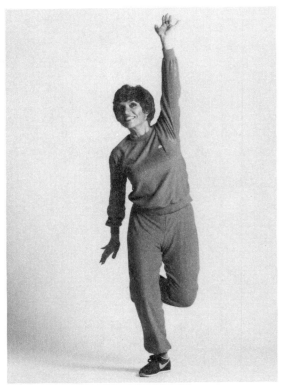

14. a. Jump onto left foot as right arm thrusts upward.

b. Repeat on other side. Rhythm is *jump*-step-step, *jump*-step-step. This is fun!

Repeat 4 times on each side.

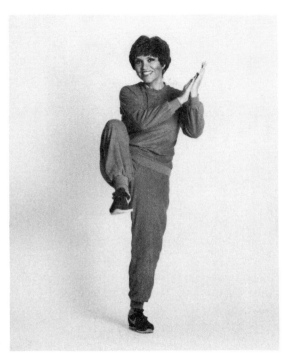 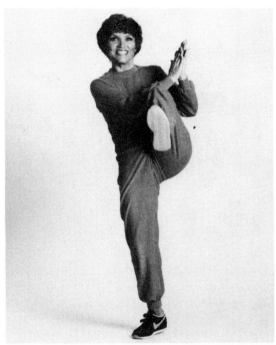

15. Step-clap and raise knee as high as you can. Start with right leg and do 8 times, alternating right and left. Are you breathing evenly? Good!

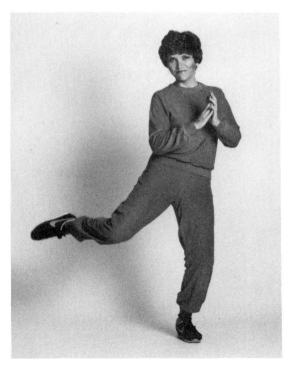 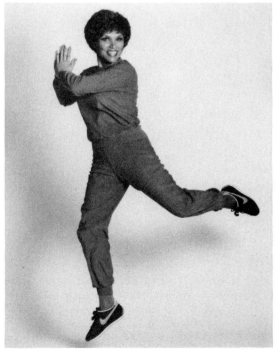

16. Now jump onto left leg and, lifting right leg behind you, clap. Repeat on other side. Do this 4 times.

129

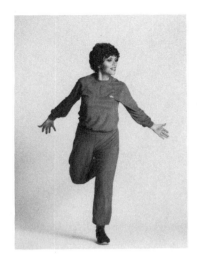 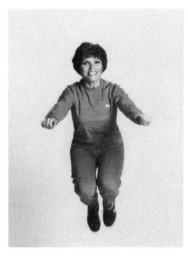 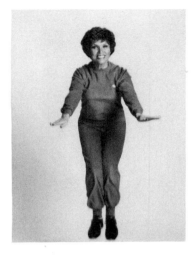

17. a. Jog in place, with hands out, for 2 counts.

b. Jump as high as you can with feet together. Swing hands forward.

c. Bring hands down as you land with knees bent.

Repeat 4 times.

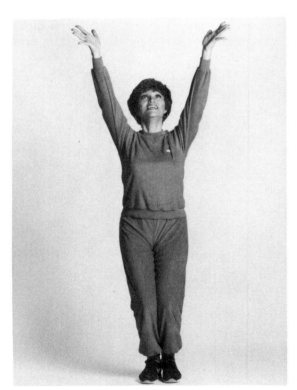

18. Swooping your arms behind you, circle arms twice and end in praise position (4 counts).

Now walk or jog in place as you take your pulse. Check the chart on page 45 or 46 to see how you're faring. Whatever you do, *don't stop moving*. Your Blessercize program always ends with a cool-down. Your heart likes it that way. Really, now, don't you feel much better already?

PART IV
THE COOL-DOWN

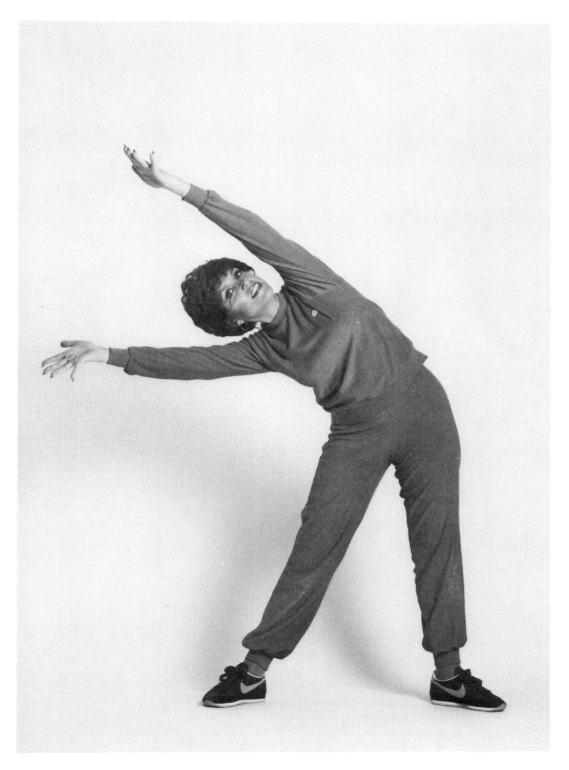

1 Pliés

Breathe deeply and evenly as your pulse rate returns to normal.

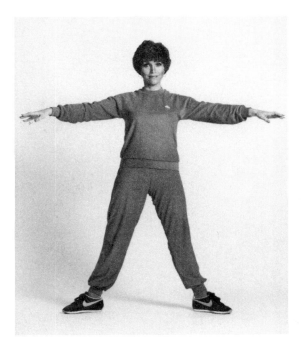

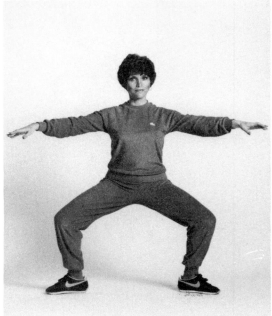

1. Standing with feet apart, arms out from sides, breathe deeply.

2. Slowly bend your knees, bringing hands down to the count of 4.

Slowly come up again to original position, bringing arms back out to sides.

Repeat 4 times.

2 Stretch and Twist

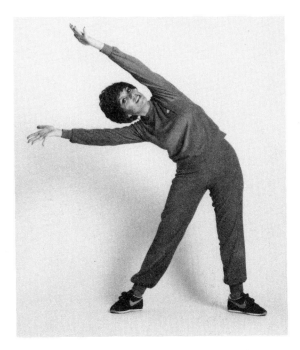 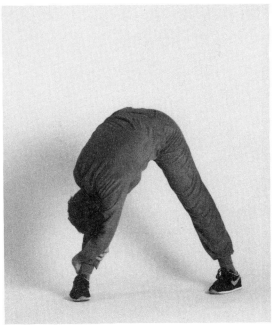

1. Same starting position as #1. Reach arms over head and bend to the right side . . .

2. . . . then twist and stretch out over your right leg, swing down, and touch nose to knee. Hold. Repeat on other side.

Do this 4 times.

Before going on to next cool-down exercise, circle your head as you did in the warm-up. (*See* page 79.) Slowly follow with shoulder circles.

3 Spaghetti

Start: Lie down flat on floor. Press small of back to floor. Breathe deeply and relax all the vertebrae and muscles.

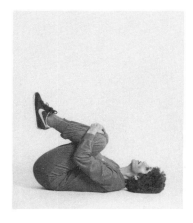
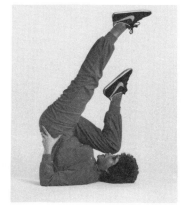
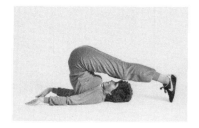

1. Now pull your knees to your chest. Feel the strength along your back.

2. Lift up your hips and support your lower back with your hands. Bicycle for the count of 8.

3. Now straighten your legs and extend them straight back, past your head, as far as possible. Try to touch the floor, keeping legs perfectly straight. (Beginners work up to it.) Hold.

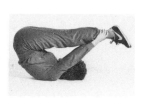
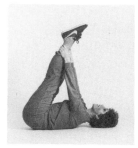
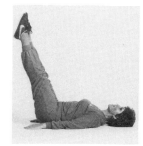
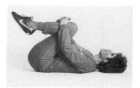

4. Grasp your ankles and hold for a count of 4.

5. Using your stomach muscles, lower your legs with control, still holding ankles.

6. With small of back on the floor, allow your legs to lower without using your hands. Use control.

7. When your legs are lowered to floor, bring knees up to your chest. Hug tightly as you totally relax.

Repeat entire sequence if you wish.

Fantastic! You did great! I'm so proud of you. I wish I were there so I could give you a big hug. Don't you feel terrific?

Let me remind you, these exercises are to be done in *progression.* Don't expect to look like a ballerina after one workout. Be good to yourself, and never, I repeat, *never,* put yourself down. Don't let me catch you telling yourself some dumb negative thing like, "I can't—" (Oh, how I hate that expression. It's positively un-Christian!)

You can do *all things* through Christ who strengthens you. There was nobody on this earth more out of shape than *me* at one time. I looked like a baby porpoise the first time I took an aerobics class. There I was, flopping around, gasping, trying to keep up with everybody else. But I refused to be discouraged. Don't you be! Resist discouragement and it will flee from you. God is on your side.

Take your recovery pulse rate five minutes after your exercise period. It should be 100 to 120 before you rest. Be sure to record in your log and count up your points.

Thank You, Jesus, for my workout today. Thank You for blessing my body and breathing life into every tissue and fiber of my being. Thank You for getting my circulation going and my heart rate up. I'm so blessed and so thankful that You have given me a body to take care of for You. Bless each muscle and cell now for Your glory. All I do and all I am is Yours. Amen.

EVERYDAY EXERCISES YOU CAN TAKE HOME, TO THE OFFICE, AND ANYWHERE

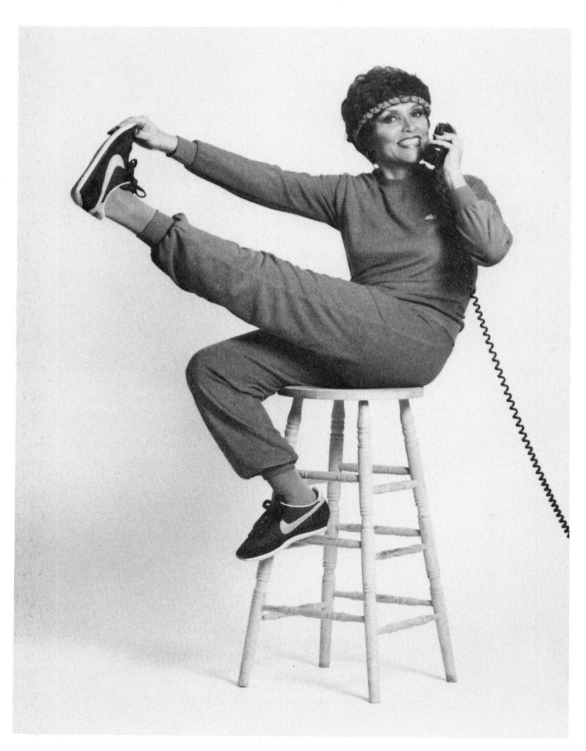

Here are some double-duty, bonus exercises you can do while working around the house or on the job, shopping, or wherever you happen to be. (A few weeks of these and laziness will be a thing of the past!)

1 On the Telephone

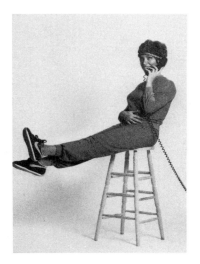 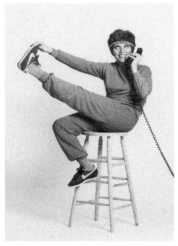 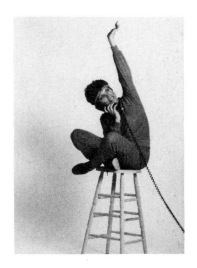

1. (Good for ankles and feet.) Sit on edge of chair. Extend legs. Make circles with your right foot, 4 clockwise and 4 counterclockwise. Pull in stomach muscles. Now flex and point your feet. Alternate up to 32 times.

2. Sit on edge of chair. Raise your leg as high as you can, keeping knee straight. Grab your toe with opposite hand. Feel the stretch along your leg and lower back. It's terrific. Repeat on opposite leg.

3. You can do these at your desk or anywhere else you're sitting down, even if you're not on the telephone. Tilting your body slightly for extra stretch, reach your left arm as high overhead as possible. Repeat 10–20 times, keeping elbow straight. Repeat with right arm. This is also good for waist.

2 Putting Away Groceries

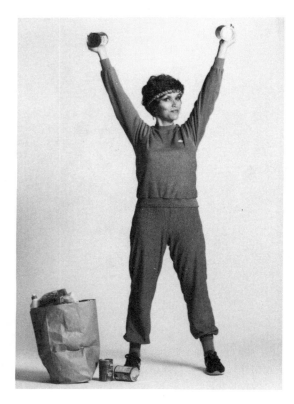
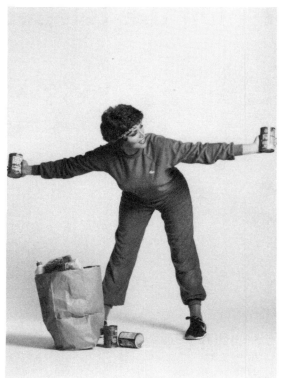

1. When you have two cans or heavy jars of the same weight, place one in each hand and raise them overhead from shoulder height, not bending your elbows. Repeat 8 times. (My friend Shirley does this one with milk containers.)

2. Bending forward from the waist, keep elbows straight and lower arms, one at a time, to your sides. Lift again to shoulder height. Repeat rapidly, 10 times each side.

In the same position, without pausing, make small circles with each arm. Rotate forward and back.

3 Raking the Leaves, Sweeping, or Vacuuming

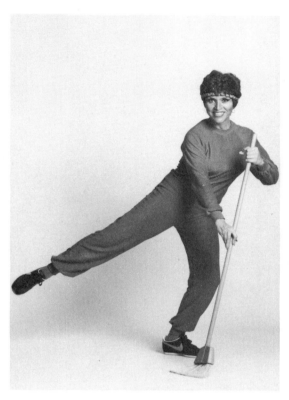 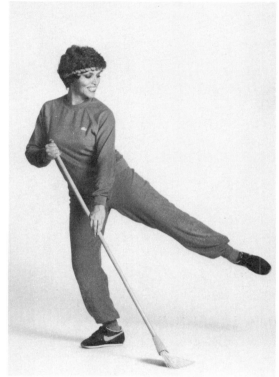

1. Stand erect, feet together. Holding handle, lunge forward on beat. Feel stretch on back of leg and hamstrings.

2. Pull weight back to starting position, keeping leg straight. Bend both knees and repeat. Alternate on both sides 4 times.

4 Doing the Laundry

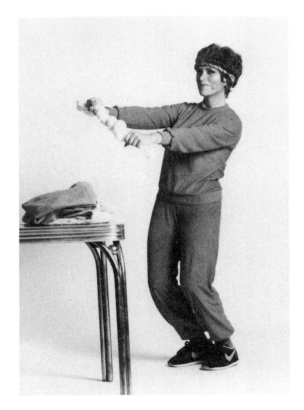

Great for your upper body and arms.

Stand leaning forward slightly, bending knees. Using an old towel, lift it shoulder level and wring it out. Tighten arms and pectorals. Reverse and twist as hard as you can. Repeat 4 times.

5 Picking Up Toys (or anything else from the floor)

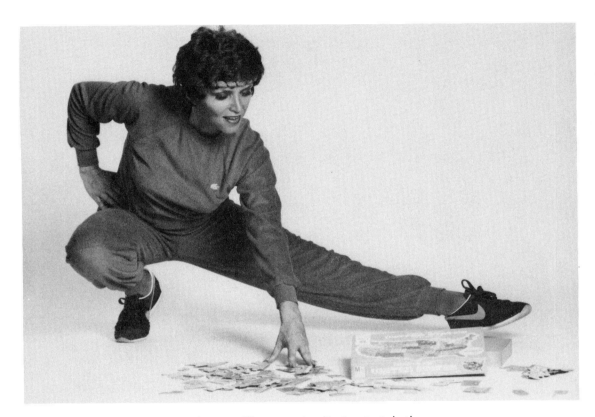

Here's a terrific opportunity to stretch those leg muscles and tendons. Place weight on bent knee. Stretch other leg out as far as it will go. Reverse sides and stretch and reach.

6 Watching TV

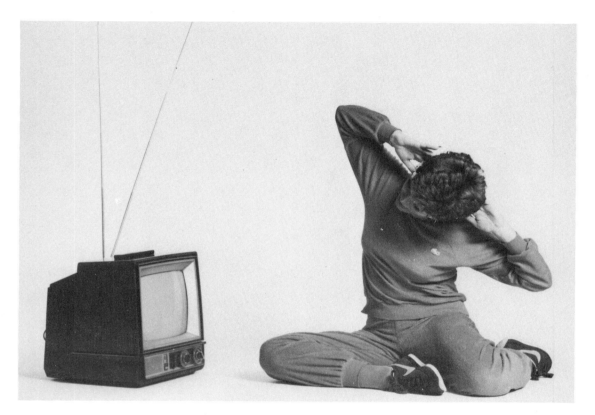

Sit on floor with right knee bent in front of you and left leg bent behind you. With hands behind head and elbows out, bend to the left. Feel the wonderful pull in your stomach, waist, and thighs. Repeat 10 times and change sides.

7 Waiting in Line

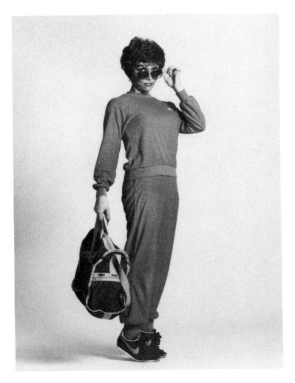 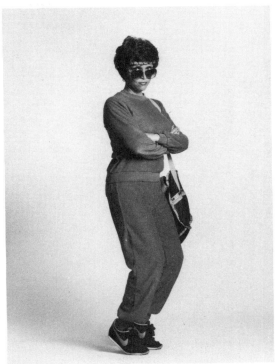

1. Think posture. Standing erect, squeeze your abdominal and buttocks muscles as tightly as you can. Raise up on your toes. Hold for a count of 10.

2. Now bend your knees, with your weight still over your toes, for a count of 10. Repeat steps 1 and 2. Guaranteed to make waiting in line more fun, and no one will even notice you are exercising.

How to Increase Muscle Strength and Keep Joints Supple and Flexible:

- Balance on one foot while putting on shoes.
- When going up stairs, take two steps at a time instead of one.
- Leave the car at home.
- While waiting for clothes to finish drying, run in place.
- When driving, sit so your knees are bent when they touch the pedals.
- Practice picking up objects from floor with your toes.

10

Maintaining for Life

The New You

After you've been on your fitness program for about three months, you will have developed habits that will stay with you. You have been working out faithfully, as well as eating to the glory of the Lord; the Word of God has been on your lips every day. You have drawn close to God and felt the breath of heaven in your body, soul, and spirit. This feeling of exhilaration and control is so magnificent that it will not be easy to fall back into the old, lazy habits you once had.

When you reach your ideal weight and are physically fit, you will feel like a new person. That's because you *will* be a new person. You'll feel as though God has given you a whole new body and a whole new life.

And you'll want to *keep* it.

Is Your Motivation Showing?

We all react differently to success. If you have been working on your fitness program with *godly motivation*, you'll handle success with godly aplomb.

Evelyn D., a dental assistant, tells how she joined a weight loss club and competed in a thirty-day weight loss contest with the rest of the members in her class. Each member put ten dollars in the kitty, so the gals meant business.

"It wasn't the idea of winning the money that motivated me," Evelyn explains. "It was an inner drive, a deep desire to do better than everybody else."

Evelyn took diuretics, water pills, and enemas to help wrench off the weight. She fasted a total of six days out of the thirty, and the rest of the month ate barely enough to keep body and soul together. Lettuce and sardines were the staple items of her diet. She said she would have cut off a leg if she thought she could manage without one. (Legs can weigh anywhere between fifteen and thirty pounds, you know.)

Evelyn lost weight, but unfortunately, not enough. An executive secretary named Ida won the kitty by three pounds, and Evelyn headed for the potato chips and a full-fledged binge. In a few days she regained every pound she had worked so hard to lose.

Motivation can be your protector or your villainous foe. Before you lose another ounce or add another sit-up to your program, give it over to the Lord to bless. "I give You this effort, Lord," tell Him. "It's all Yours. I am an achiever because I achieve through the power of the Holy Spirit."

If you grab the rope of human pride and swing with it, you're bound to land in the bushes of failure.

Handling Attention

Handling attention will be something you might want to prepare yourself for. Your friends may ooh and ah, but then again, they may not. A fat, dumpy person is no threat to anyone else's ego. (If you don't believe me, how many times have you resisted jealousy when you saw an overweight, out-of-shape person?)

Aristotle wrote these words twenty-three hundred years ago: "Beauty is a greater recommendation than any letter of introduction." Things haven't really changed much since Aristotle's day. In an article by Dr. K. Dion in the *Journal of Personality and Social Psychology*, he tells of a test he made where he showed college women photographs of children who had allegedly misbehaved. Some of the children were physically attractive and others were not. When the misbehavior was a severe one, the beautiful

children were given the benefit of the doubt. Respondents tended to disregard the behavior of the attractive children, whereas less attractive children who committed the same act were called maladjusted and deviant. Even children themselves are aware of these differences. Dion has found that children as young as three years old will prefer pretty children to homely ones.

Studies have shown that the highly attractive person is more likely to be recommended for hiring on a job interview, or to have his or her work evaluated favorably. These studies powerfully demonstrate the extent to which we rely on physical appearance in making judgments of other people.

Back in 1937, sociologist W. W. Walker explained that being seen with an attractive person of the opposite sex brings a great deal of self-prestige. The underlying feeling is that the other person's attractiveness will somehow "rub off." In making these choices, people combine information about personal attractiveness with their own judgment of being accepted.

People with strong leadership qualities fare better if they are attractive. In the Old Testament, when the people wanted a king, they chose the most handsome man they could find. Tall, handsome Saul was the one the people wanted. There were probably a lot of qualified homely men around, but Saul *looked* good, so he got the job.

Mary D., who lost twenty pounds, got herself in shape and became the real Mary. She told us after a Fun to Be Fit class one day, "I've been going to the same service station with my car for years. They have never given me any preferential treatment. In fact, I have had to *beg* for prompt service in the past. Yesterday I brought the car in and the very same mechanic greeted me as if I were Princess Diana and my car was the Royal Driving Machine. He was actually *nice* to me!"

When you receive favorable attention from others, tell the Lord Jesus, "Lord, I refuse to get proud because I look good." Just remember, King David looked good. Daniel looked good. Queen Esther was a veritable beauty queen. Sarah, wife of Abraham, was a notoriously beautiful woman, and Ruth was no schlepp, either.

You have the right to look good, too. You are a *Christian.* You're a light set on a hill. Go on out there representing Christ, and let your light shine.

The attention you receive, whether negative or positive, belongs to the Lord. When I wrote the life story of singer Tom Netherton, I observed how he handled attention. Tom is a handsome fellow and the girls literally flock around him. In fact, girls even write to me because I wrote a book about handsome Tom. They want me to introduce them to him.

Tom told me that when he auditioned for "The Lawrence Welk Show," he prayed earnestly, "If I can glorify *You,* Jesus, by being on television, then that's what I want." Tom's desire was to glorify the Lord, not bring fame and attention to himself. God honored Tom's prayer, and Tom is now a celebrated Christian television-and-concert performer. He leads many people to Jesus Christ every year. His love of God is an inspiration to countless people. Tom also exercises daily and keeps fit by playing tennis and using a stationary bicycle.

Tom looks good. So can you.

And you can *stay* that way without becoming proud.

Four Basic Keys to Maintaining

Add new exercises to your program

I have chosen the most effective exercises out of hundreds for this book.

Please add your own to the ones I've given you here. Your muscles need two weeks of doing the same exercises to develop strength in the areas you're working on, but after six weeks, you can add new ones and new progressions.

See yourself as God sees you

"I have loved thee with an everlasting love: therefore with lovingkindness have I drawn thee . . ." (Jeremiah 31:3). You are a new you because of God's love for you. He has helped you, guided you, blessed you. He has shown you *He* is love and, as He is, so are you (1 John 4:17). He loved you even before you got in shape, and He always will love you. Tell yourself you are representing *Him* with the new you, body, soul, and spirit. God is looking upon you with infinite love and tenderness. Say out loud every day, "Lord, I am loved and cherished by You and I have Your Spirit within me. That means I *will* stay on my lifetime fitness program. I am never alone. You are the strength of my life."

Schedule your exercise time

Exercise will never again be an option in your life. It is a permanent appointment on your daily schedule. When you schedule your week, schedule your fitness time, including exercising, aerobics, and aerobic activities.

Keep fitness wise

This means keeping informed. I highly suggest reading books on fitness, joining exercise classes, buying health food recipe books, and learning all you can about health and fitness. This will keep your interest spurred and your mind continually fresh with fitness tips and information. You will be less likely to make an excuse to fall prey to the old attack of the "Wild Munchies" if you're regularly reading about health and nutrition. Also, you're not likely to skip your exercise time if you're busy learning all you can about exercise through books and periodicals. Kathryn Lance, who wrote *Getting Strong* and *Running for Health and Beauty,* says she subscribes to *Runner's World* magazine and saves articles for those times when she feels her general interest in her own running program is flagging.

Your Right to Be Fit

The reason Christians haven't been concerned about physical fitness is that we somehow think anything to do with the body is "carnal." Overeating and slothfulness is far more carnal than employing self-discipline and effort to be fit and healthy, if our motives are for the glory of the Lord.

You are not being carnal if you are taking care of the body God gave you. Neglect and self-destruction is carnal. The very word *carnal* pertains to a person's passions and appetites. It means not spiritual, but merely human. Carnality is characterized by sensuality of the body, and fleshly pleasures. But the Apostle Paul said, "And they that are Christ's have crucified the flesh with the affections and lusts" (Galatians 5:24).

The definition of *physical fitness,* according to the *Physical Fitness Research Digest,* published by the President's Council on Physical Fitness and Sports, is "the ability to carry out daily tasks with vigor and alertness, without undue fatigue, and with ample energy to enjoy leisure-time pursuits and to meet unusual situations and unforeseen emergencies." We can safely say, then, that physical fitness gives you the ability to live at your utmost level of health and vitality. Fitness enables you to be mentally, emotionally, and physically alert and sound.

The words "Let not sin therefore reign in your mortal body . . ." (Romans 6:12), mean to the lazy, slothful person that he needs to decide who is Lord over his body. How often we think serving the Lord has nothing to do with being healthy or physically fit. When we read the words in Romans 12:1, that we are to present our bodies a living sacrifice, holy, acceptable unto God, we also read that this is our *reasonable* service. God is showing us that it is only right and natural that we should present our bodies to Him, that we might be in top shape for His use.

If you were to hire somebody to work for you in your company, would you choose the one who was glowing with health, energy, and strength, or would you choose one who preferred to sit all day in lethargy and sullenness? Though both employees may love you and be dedicated to you and the company, which one would be of the most service to you?

You are a person fit for the Master's use now. Say out loud, "In Him I am complete."

Jesus said that He came to give you life and to give it to you more abundantly (John 10:10). This tells us that we have a right to an abundance of God's life as Christians. The word *zoe,* found in the New Testament 130 times, means "life." This life is God's own life, and this life you have a right to.

The life of God lives within you because you are filled with His Spirit. *Zoe* is God Himself, and you have within you the life of God. Even if you think you could never be physically fit, you can grasp the words "All things are possible to them who believe" (*see* Mark 9:23). You are filled with God's own life. You have a right to a full and abundant life and can expect to be *complete* in Christ (Colossians 2:10).

By receiving enough of the life of

God, you are made more than a conqueror, spirit, soul, and body.

Call it what you will, obesity by any other name is just plain fat and out of shape. We get that way because of neglect. What could be more carnal?

The Christian Yo-Yo Syndrome

It has been proven that fitness gives us a sense of self-esteem. When you feel good about yourself, you can be freer to accept and recognize the needs in other people's lives. If you have become physically fit through the right motives, your desire is to love and to serve.

A wrong motive for the Christian is a "religious" approach to fitness. Religiosity is not the same as having a relationship with Jesus Christ. A religious spirit approaches a fitness program with a condemned heart looking for absolution. That person may emerge three months later with a new, fit body, but if he or she has been motivated by a religious attitude toward fitness, an insidious binge might be lurking around the corner.

That's because the condemned heart is the primary manipulator, with confession and absolution in close pursuit. The person trapped in the "Christian Yo-Yo Syndrome" develops a legion of ego injuries, all of which revolve around guilt, confession, and absolution. This is a violent insult to personal integrity. It is essential to understand that *becoming physically fit is not punishment*. It is an honor and a joy. That is why I have called this book *Fun to Be Fit*.

Think enjoyment. If you find yourself interpolating self-criticism and bitter demands into your fitness program, do as Juan Perón advised: "Answer violence with violence!"

Take an adamant stand against self-condemnation, putting on the full armor of God. Those stinging barbs of guilt stabbing at tissues of your self-worth are not heaven inspired.

Part of my job as a therapist is to teach my patients who have overeating problems to make eating *fun* again. The unrealistic pressures the world puts on us to be thin makes us feel guilty if we enjoy food. How many times have you heard, "This tastes so good, it must be a sin"?

The weight loss and exercise programs which have failed for you in the past may have been counterproductive because there was little attention paid to your psychological need for self-approval. Failure and guilt go together like toast and butter. Excuse the analogy. You need to approve of yourself, yet you like cherry pie. How on earth can you eat cherry pie and *still* like yourself?

So you don't eat the pie, but then one day you have an emotional setback, and you have an *affaire d'amour* with the cherry pie, eating the entire thing. Such a binge could put as many as fifteen thousand calories into your precious body. Getting the extra pounds off is the purge. There you are again.

The solution is to grant yourself a piece of pie once in a while, if that's what you want. Plan for it and *enjoy* it. Getting fit is not a religion; it's a joyful expression of our love for God.

A patient of mine, Heidi, lost twenty-five pounds and has kept it off for the last two years. I set her program up to include some of her favorite high-calorie foods. She rebelled at first, accustomed to her binge-purge yo-yo syndrome. I was insistent.

I threatened her one day with, "If you don't have spaghetti and meatballs and garlic bread for dinner tonight, don't come back to see me."

Heidi's program allowed for occasional indulgences. So can yours. Bless yourself with discipline and plan for those times when you'll want to eat something you've thought of as "forbidden." That way you won't sneak into the kitchen in the dead of the night, as Heidi had in the past, and attack the refrigerator to gobble down leftover cold spaghetti out of a bowl, picking the cold meatballs out with your fingers.

Some rules of thumb to follow:

1. *Schedule your indulgences.* On the day you are going to have that extra-calorie meal, eat less for breakfast and lunch. (*Don't* skip meals. Remember your blood sugar. You don't want to eat the house out, do you?) Plan ahead and then stick to the plan. Perhaps you will want to reduce your intake the following day, too.

2. *Weigh yourself.* Keep a check on how much your indulgences cost. Maybe that fifteen-hundred-calorie-splurge meal was more than your plan could take. You don't *ever* want to starve yourself for overeating.

3. *Stick to your exercise program.* Just because you had a big lunch doesn't mean you can skip your workout. Exercise no matter what, but not right after eating. Wait a couple of hours, but exercise. *Always* exercise.

SAMPLE CALORIE EXPENDITURES

ACTIVITY	CALORIES BURNED PER HOUR
Jogging	600
Swimming (moderate crawl)	600
Tennis (singles)	500
Cross-Country Skiing	1300
Bicycling (moderate pace)	450
Tennis (doubles)	400
Bowling (very actively)	400
Volleyball	350
Walking (vigorously)	350
Golf	300
Floor Mopping (vigorously)	300
Walking (moderately)	200
Ironing (strenuously)	200
Typing	145
Driving	130
Singing	125
Brushing Hair	100
Talking on the Telephone	50
Jumping Rope (80 turns per minute)	620
Food Shopping	190

(Figures are based on a body weight of approximately 125 pounds, with more calories expended for more weight and less calories if you weigh less than 125.)

11

Kingdom Fitness

What It Is

A pastor friend of mine in California lost forty pounds reading *Free to Be Thin*. He is now engaging in a daily Fun to Be Fit program. He tells everyone who will listen about the newfound energy he's gained and the change that fitness has made in his life as a minister. He is no longer tired and fatigued at the end of the day, and he feels better than he has in ten years. His congregation is benefiting from their pastor's new strength and energy. Because he feels better and has more vitality, his people have a healthier, happier leader. Many of them have lost weight and are getting in shape, too. Being in control of your body will not only bless you but others will benefit, too, because you will have more time, energy, and optimism to give.

My own pastor is a picture of fitness and runs a couple of miles every day. In a church of over one thousand mem-

bers, he always has time for the people of his congregation. He has the energy of several men and is enormously admired and respected. These pastors, as well as several of my other friends in various ministries around the world, are avid proponents of what I call "Kingdom Fitness."

For the kingdom of God is not meat
and drink; but righteousness, and peace,
and joy in the Holy Ghost.

Romans 14:17

According to the Amplified Version of the Bible, the Kingdom of God is having and being in that state which makes a person acceptable to God. It's also the peace within us that cannot be disturbed, no matter what. It is the joy of the Holy Spirit, so sublime and other-worldly, that all we do and are becomes a celebration of God.

For he that in these things serveth Christ is acceptable to God, and approved of men.

Romans 14:18

151

You were born to be a citizen of the Kingdom of God. You were born to serve here, live here, and invest your total being here. Righteousness, peace, and joy are your rights as a citizen of the Kingdom of God. You inherited them as yours when you said yes to Jesus Christ as your Savior, and you appropriate them as you learn more of God every day.

The above verse tells us that we are acceptable to God. How many years have you clamored for acceptance of *people?* This verse tells us that we are acceptable to God and therefore are approved of by people. Fitness is not the Kingdom of God, no; righteousness, peace, and joy in the Holy Spirit are. But you cannot experience the fullness of these things as a sickly, hurting, tired, depressed, nervous, overweight, irritable person. Knowing that your body is the temple of God (1 Corinthians 3:16), and your life is hid in Christ (Colossians 3:3), who is being formed in you (Galatians 4:19), you have the *right* to take what's yours and to expect God to use you.

Your life will be an example from now on. You won't have to say a word about fitness—your life will show that you are a person who has learned self-discipline and faithful adherence to a fitness program. You can help those who need the Lord in this area of their lives by proving it can be done.

We then that are strong ought to bear the infirmities of the weak, and not to please ourselves.

Romans 15:1

The Apostle Paul understood the seriousness of his relationship to God and the ministry given to him. Paul lived a long life and he said, "I keep under my body, and bring it into subjection: lest that by any means, when I have preached to others, I myself should be a castaway" (1 Corinthians 9:27).

There is widespread interest in diet and exercise among the cults. Yoga is a good example. It was developed as an Eastern religious expression and is practiced in this country today, even in the churches. Christians are going to yoga classes to trim and tone their bodies, performing the pagan exercises and even the positions of prayer and devotion to Hindu gods right in their own church basements.

Many Christians interested in self-defense and martial-arts activities may be nonplussed to know that practices such as karate, aikido, judo, and kendo have their origins in demon worship. If you are engaged in these practices, be sure you understand the spiritual danger involved. You may be opening yourself up to some negative, even horrible, influences.

Cultish zeal for diet and exercise usually ends up with something missing. The devil is not dumb enough to allow people perfect health. The difference between you and the non-Christian health-food aficionado is that you have the wisdom of God within you through Jesus Christ. You resist the devil and his crazy health claims, and follow the truth.

A diet in point is the macrobiotic diet, desperately lacking in protein and calcium. George Ohsawa, the originator of macrobiotic food and author of *The Unique Principle,* upholds the yang and yin theory, which is "like a flying arrow out of reach of those who want to possess it." The point he makes is that once you grasp hold of the flying arrow, it is no longer flying. (To some people this is a philosophical revelation.) The yang and yin philosophy states that the universe is composed of the movement of two basic forces, male and female, contraction and expansion, animal and vegetable, fire and water, and on and on down to sweet and sour.

God never meant food to be a religion. Vegetarianism, macrobiotic eating, and other "religiously oriented" programs are usually lacking as ideal. Many people have died on the macrobiotic food plan. The exercises of yoga and other Eastern occult physical endeavors are grounded and founded on demon worship, and the Christian should stay away from them.

Now therefore, if ye will obey my voice indeed, and keep my covenant, then ye shall be a peculiar treasure unto me above all people: for all the earth is mine.

Exodus 19:5

The Only Recipe in This Book

I am going to tell you about my Super-Dynamite Smoothie, a drink so delicious, you won't believe it's healthy—a definite Kingdom taste thrill.

I've shared this recipe with lots of people, important people—like my mom, the gang down at the Christian Center for Counseling and Fitness, my daughter's math teacher—and let me tell you, I've gotten nothing but raves. It is a total hit.

This drink could very well change your taste buds. I tell you, you'll never drink another ugly ice-cream milk shake or malted again if you can have a Super-Dynamite Smoothie.

To begin with, let a few bananas get real ripe, not a speck of green on them. Let them get dark yellow and brown. Then break them into three or four chunks, put them in a small plastic bag, and freeze them. I freeze a dozen or so at a time.

Recipe for One Smoothie

1 frozen banana
1 cup apple juice
1 tablespoon protein powder

Put it all in a blender, blend, and there you have it. Ambrosia. It's thick, like a milk shake, and delicious. For variety add any of the following alone or with other fruits:

strawberries
blueberries
peaches
apricots
pineapple

You may use any fruit juice in place of apple juice. Orange is fabulous; pineapple sublime; grape delicious. Combination juices are especially good, as is any natural, unsweetened juice. You may want to add some honey for sweetener, and if you're a vitamin lover, one or more of the following:

natural yeast (only 1 teaspoon)
unprocessed bran (1 tablespoon)
1 tablespoon safflower oil
1 raw egg
1 tablespoon wheat germ

Drink this Super-Dynamite Smoothie every day and you'll make your "sweet tooth" very happy. (What on earth is a sweet tooth? I know if I had one, I'd probably eat it.)

My Super-Dynamite Smoothie is not one of those health drinks you plug your nose to drink and then shudder for six minutes after you take the last swallow. I serve this for company. My children serve it to their friends after school. It's an especially great summer drink. Just remember, you can go wild with creativity making the Smoothie. Frozen banana and apple juice are your basic ingredients; then you add to that. It makes a delightful Christmas drink by adding frozen cranberries and a little honey to the basic recipe.

Your Spiritual Vitamins

The following spiritual vitamins are in tract form, distributed by my ministry. Over twenty thousand people have these in their Bibles, notebooks, and pockets. I am constantly receiving letters from people who tell me how their spiritual vitamins have helped them. Use them on your Fun to Be Fit program.

Repeat three times daily and at bedtime.

- "I am complete in Jesus Christ, who is the head of all principality and power" (see Colossians 2:10).
- I am in Him complete, made full, and have come to fullness of life.
- "The same spirit that raised up Jesus from the dead dwells in me!" (see Romans 8:11).
- "And greater is He that is in me than he that is in the world" (see I John 4:4).
- I am of God—I belong to Him—and I have defeated the enemy and his agents because Jesus Christ, who lives in me by the power of His Holy Spirit, is greater, mightier, and more powerful than the devil who is in the world.
- "I am submitted to God and in the mighty name of Jesus, I resist the devil and he flees from me" (see James 4:7).
- "Jesus is my redeemer. I am redeemed from sin and I am also redeemed from sickness. Just as I resist sin, I resist sickness in the name of Jesus. If disease attaches itself to my body, I have an advocate, Jesus Christ, to heal, forgive, and cleanse me. *By His stripes I am healed and made whole"* (see 1 Peter 2:24).
- "God has given me a spirit of power and love and of a calm and well-balanced mind. I do not receive a spirit of fear, timidity, or cowardice" (see 2 Timothy 1:7).
- I choose to prosper in all I do unto God. I choose to receive health, financial well-being, emotional stability, and happiness as a redeemed child of the living God. I refuse negativity, doubt, fear, sickness, and strife of any kind in my life.
- "I choose to live a life of abundance because He came that I may have and enjoy life, and have it in abundance to the full, till it overflows" (see John 10:10).
- "I suffer no lack because the Lord is my Shepherd, I *shall not lack"* (see Psalms 23:1).

Surely goodness and mercy are following me all the days of my life, as I live pressed tightly to God forever.

See Psalms 23:6

12

A Beautiful Tomorrow

Something beautiful in my life
Something beautiful,
He made something beautiful in my life.

The words of that song go on to say, "All my confusion, He understood, / all I had to offer Him was brokenness and strife / but He made something beautiful in my life."

Francis MacNutt, in his book *Healing*, says that Jesus came to do two basic things:

1. Positive: To give us a new life, a loving relationship of union with His Father and with Himself, through the Holy Spirit.
2. In relation to the obstacles to new life: To heal and free (save) us from all those sick elements in the human personality that need to be transformed so that the new life may freely enter in.

Jesus came to heal those whose spirits were sick and needed deliverance and forgiveness. He also healed those people who had lame bodies, who were blind, dying, and leprous. Every time a sick person came to Jesus in faith, He healed that person. He did not divide man, as we are inclined to do, into a soul to be saved and healed and a body that is to suffer and remain weak or sick. Jesus Christ came to save us, spirit, soul, and body. Jesus saw us as whole persons. It is a pagan view of the universe stemming from Platonic, Stoic, and Manichaean sources, that the body is an encumbrance and an enemy to the spirit. The Bible does not tell us to regard the body as an enemy, but to celebrate its goodness. The Bible teaches us to avoid the *sins* of the body, not the body itself.

Fitness and Your Age

Frances Sackerman ran her first mile in 1972 when she was forty-three years old. She built up systematically the duration and intensity of her runs, and began entering 10K races. She won the San Francisco Diet Pepsi 10K, setting a new American record in her age group when she was fifty years old by running it in 41:28. She is still running and at the age of fifty-two, she is going strong. Runners in their forties, fifties, sixties, and over have laid to rest the old mistaken notion that the golden years are a time for sinking into the rocking chair. My Great-Uncle Fred, who is in his eighties, is not about to sink into his rocking chair. In fact, he doesn't even own one. He does, however, own a stationary bicycle and a slant board. He sees no reason to stop being fit—ever.

Jack La Lanne is no spring chicken, and he is in better shape than many of the twenty-year-olds who come into his health spas. The great modern dance artist Martha Graham danced well into her eighties. There is no reason for anybody to stop being active simply because of his or her advanced age. If you are between forty and eighty, and you are experiencing listlessness, tiredness, and a general lack of energy, instead of going to bed earlier, add some exercise to your life. Check with your doctor, read this book again, and expect God to do something good for you.

Any exercise plan you engage in should work on the basis of an easy start and gradual progression. As your physical fitness improves, you can increase your work load. "Something beautiful in my life" can be your song at any age.

Walking

Walking can be an enormous source of joy and discovery in your life, as well as a great benefit to your health. According to the *Official YMCA Physical Fitness Handbook*, you *especially* should be walking every day if you have high blood pressure, are overweight, score poorly on cardiovascular fitness tests, have orthopedic problems, or are over sixty years of age.

Schedule a time to walk every day and begin with a warm-up. Even though walking is in itself a warm-up, it uses the same muscles as jogging, so warm up before setting out. (*See* warm-up exercises on pages 77 through 87.

Pace yourself to start slowly and walk only a short distance, say, around the block. Gradually increase the distance as you shorten the time you walk it to adjust to increased energy output and muscle exertion. Breathe deeply. Enjoy the scenery. This is a wonderful opportunity to meditate on the Word of God and pray for someone who is not as healthy and fit as you are.

Something Beautiful Even Away From Home

When you're traveling, bring along your sneakers and running clothes, a jump rope (one of those plastic-link kind, not the one in your children's toy box) and a light mat or beach towel for the floor. You can exercise in your motel or hotel room with no problem at all. It's always fun to run in a strange town, too. My friend Doris Whitesell of Chicago has told me some of her most wonderful experiences have been running when she has been traveling and visiting her family in Sweden. She told me how she ran the hills, countryside, and small villages even in the night, when her days had gotten too busy to run. The feeling she received was one of exhilaration. Doris also bicycles everywhere she goes, and takes week-long bicycle trips with her family in the summertime in Vermont.

Ann Kiemel, in her book *I'm Running to Win,* tells how she continued her running program while on her speaking tours. She arose in the morning while it was still dark, took a taxi ten miles out of town, and ran back to the hotel where she was staying. Then she showered and dressed for the day. She says so poignantly, "If we could just fall in love with Jesus. If only we could love Him so much that every day we would be unwilling to give less than our best. . . ."

Vacations can do you in faster than you can say, "Which way to the dining room?" There's something about those hotel smorgasbords that brings out the maniac in even the staunchest dieter. And after a day of lying on the beach or watching a bobber at the end of your fishing line on the water, chocolate ice cream begins to take on a new meaning to you. You suddenly forget how to spell grapefruit. You remember the pastry of last night's smorgasbord. Thoughts of the fish fry tonight send goose bumps up your back.

Vacations are no time to vacation from your eating program and your exercise program. One binge can make you feel so guilty, you won't exercise that day. How can you? You're suffering from acid indigestion, bloated stomach, food hangover, and a severe case of guilt.

Dr. Frank Katch, head of the exercise science department of the University of Massachusetts, says, "The difference between overweight people and normal weight people is not only how much they eat, but how much they move." On vacation, it almost seems a sin to move. The only moving you want to do is toward the dessert cart at lunch. You snicker cleverly as you eat and tell your friends or family, "I'm checking to see if anything's poisoned."

Why not take a "fitness vacation" this year? Plan for you and your family to go somewhere you can run together in the morning, swim together before lunch, play tennis in the afternoon, and eat nu-

tritiously all the while. You will feel terrific and come back home far more rested than if you had spent your entire vacation sleeping. Check with your travel agent about the many recreational places you can go that will enhance your aerobics program. Riding tour buses, horseback riding, going to the movies, and being the first in line at the breakfast smorgasbord are not aerobic activities. One of the favorite family vacations among my friends is skiing. Spending a week flying down the white slopes, with the wind rushing at their faces and their hearts filled with the free and euphoric sensation of flying, is something they look forward to all year long. Skiing is a good aerobic exercise. A daily workout, coupled with some regular walking, and you will stay fit for anything.

Some Final Tips

Continue to exercise to Scripture

When doing any exercise, use Scripture as your counting system. Do leg raises to the Twenty-third Psalm, for instance. Do two Twenty-third Psalms on each side. Do fifteen Mark 11:24s like this: Recite the verse and at the end say, "One." Then repeat it again, and at the end add, "Two!" And on you go until you have completed the set.

"Think on these things"

Be in control of your thoughts as you exercise. While running, for example, plan what you'll eat that day. If you plan your menus at this time, chances are you'll choose only healthy foods, like salads, fruit, and protein. I can't imagine running while dreaming about eating heavy, fattening food.

Focus on "something beautiful"

Envision God at work in every area of your life. Imagine your prayers answered. Take this opportunity to pray for lost loved ones and people who are hurting, in trouble, and in need of your prayers. But don't just pray, "Lord, bless them." Concentrate on seeing that prayer answered. Lift up your vision to the Lord for Him to see. Claim the answers and repeat a Scripture which pertains to the person or situation you are praying about. Your exercise time can be a glorious adventure with the Lord every day. Don't expect anything less.

He is making something beautiful of your life.

Reward yourself

In the past, your rewards were not really rewards at all, but punishers. As your daily log points increase and you reach and maintain your goals, be sure to reward yourself regularly. Your rewards could include an extra Blessercize, a new pair of sweat socks with your initials stitched on the sides, some marvelous bath oil, a new hairstyle, giving more of your time to your church, or buying a new Christian book for yourself to read after you exercise. God wants to reward you.

Your new body is a reward in itself, but you can give yourself a happy bonus reward or two. God loves to give good things to His children. He loves to bless you. He loves to say, "Well done, good and faithful servant" (see Matthew 25:21).

I believe that's what He's saying right now.

> O Lord,
>   you have
>   freed me
> from my bonds
> and I will
> serve you
>   forever.
> Psalms 116:16 TLB

The Fun to Be Fit program plus additional Blessercize by Marie Chapian is available on cassette by sending $6.95 (includes postage) to:

Fun to Be Fit
Christian Center for Counseling and Fitness
P. O. Box 16655
San Diego, CA 92116

California residents add 6% sales tax.

BIBLIOGRAPHY

Backus, William, and Chapian, Marie. *Telling Yourself the Truth.* Minneapolis: Bethany House Publishers, 1980.

Batten, Jack. *The Complete Jogger.* New York: Harcourt Brace Jovanovich, Inc., 1977.

Bevan, James, M.D. *The Simon & Schuster Handbook of Anatomy and Physiology.* New York: Simon & Schuster, Inc., 1979.

Bosworth, F. F. *Christ the Healer.* Old Tappan, New Jersey: Fleming H. Revell Company, 1973.

Chapian, Marie. *Free to Be Thin.* Minneapolis: Bethany House Publishers, 1979.

Cooper, Kenneth H., M.D. *Aerobics.* New York: Bantam Books, Inc., 1972.

————. *The New Aerobics.* New York: M. Evans & Company Inc., 1970.

Dion, K. "Attractiveness and Evaluation of Children's Transgressions." *Journal of Personality and Social Psychology,* 1972, 24, 207–213.

————. "The Incentive Value of Physical Attractiveness for Young Children." *Personality and Social Psychology Bulletin,* 1977, 3, 67–70.

Dion, K., Berscheid, E., and Walster, E. "What Is Beautiful Is Good." *Journal of Personality and Social Psychology,* 1972, 24, 285–290.

Editors of Runner's World. *The Complete Runner.* Mountain View, California: Anderson World, Inc., 1974.

Fixx, James F. *The Complete Book of Running.* New York: Random House, Inc., 1977.

Heller, Alfred L., M.D. *Your Body, His Temple.* Nashville: Thomas Nelson, Inc., 1981.

Kiemel, Ann. *I'm Running to Win.* Wheaton, Illinois: Tyndale House Publishers, 1980.

Lance, Kathryn, *Running for Health and Beauty.* New York: Bantam Books, Inc., 1978.

————. *Getting Strong.* New York: Bobbs-Merrill Company, Inc., 1978.

MacNutt, Francis, O.P. *Healing.* New York: Bantam Books, Inc., 1977.

Myers, Clayton R. *The Official YMCA Physical Fitness Book.* New York: Popular Library, Inc., 1975.

Nyad, Diana, and Hogan, Candice L. *Basic Training for Women.* New York: Crown Publishers, Inc., 1981.

Otis, Don. *Keeping Fit.* Medford, Oregon: Omega Publications, 1979.

Royal Canadian Air Force Exercise Plans for Physical Fitness. 1976.

Shelton, Herbert M., Ph.D. *Exercise.* Bridgeport, Connecticut: Natural Hygiene, 1971.

Sorensen, Jacki, and Bruns, Bill. *Aerobic Dancing.* New York: Rawson, Wade Publishers, Inc., 1979.